Winning the Inc

Simple, no-nonsense weight loss for grown ups

Authors

Paul Lonsdale & Ann Hirst

2ND Edition

Published by

Get Physical Ltd

Copyright

Disclaimer

This book is solely for educational and informational purposes only and is not intended as an accompaniment or replacement to medical advice. It should not be used to diagnose or treat any illness, metabolic disorder or health problem.

As with all materials related to health, exercise and diet, you must first consult your doctor, physician or health care provider before implementing changes to your life style.

The authors make no representation or warranties of any kind with regard to the completeness, accuracy or safety of the contents of this book.

The authors accept no liability of any kind for losses or damages caused or alleged to be caused directly, or indirectly, from using the information contained herein

WARNING

This book contains graphic depictions of common sense. It is not suitable for anyone who prefers to keep their head stuck firmly where the sun doesn't shine!

Table of contents

Preface

In one way or another, we've spent our entire lives in the health and fitness industry. In 2002, we opened Get Physical, our personal training company in Sheffield. Then, in 2014 - after years of writing articles for a variety of magazines - we published our first book: Dump the Diets, Ditch the Scales, Drop the Inches. However, earlier this year (2018), we had a revamp and expanded to move online with a brand-new website under the banner of 'Winning the Inch War'. So, we sat down, rewrote and renamed the original book to fall in line with our new venture. In the process, we've cut out a lot, making it more concise and relevant to the reader (it seems ironic that a book about weight loss should go on a diet).

So, before we get started, we'd just to mention that this book is a jointly written effort from both of us, hence the continual use of the pronoun 'we' throughout the book. Although I'm the one who puts the words on the page, I can get a bit carried away with the sciencey-bits, so Ann is the one who then puts them in the right order! Without Ann (who is the type of woman that could teach common sense at Cambridge) this book would be full of phrases such as *'calcium ion exchange across the sarcoplasmic reticulum'*, or *'phospholipid bi-layer cell membrane'*.

We'd also like to point out that this is a self-published book, so please excuse any typos and inconsistency of grammar, etc. I think I've finally managed to break the spelling and grammar checker on Word 2016 because it no longer underlines any errors, but just waves a white flag!

Finally, it's impossible to cover every single dietary and training option, so we've kept to the basics and added lots more meal options, recipes and training videos to our website. You can find us at **www.getphysical.co.uk** and if you have any questions, please don't hesitate to get in touch. You can drop us an email at **info@getphyscial.co.uk** and our phone number is **0114 2666433** (our full contact details can be found at the end of the book).

By the way, this is not a novel, so please feel free to read it in any order that you wish.

PART 1:
DUMP THE DIETS, DITCH THE SCALES, DROP THE INCHES

'You don't need to live like a saint to have the body of an angel'
Paul & Ann

Chapter 1:
Weight loss for grown ups

'Dieting is like living in a world of soup, armed only with a fork'
Paul & Ann

Without a shadow of a doubt, weight control can be such a struggle. Yet strangely enough most people understand why they gain weight, they just don't understand why they can't lose it. We've never had a client that's claimed, "I don't get it. I went to bed resembling a Greek God and woke up looking like Buddha! I must have had a visit from the Fat Fairy*again".

But, why is it so hard to shift the weight?

Well, there are many explanations. A restrictive diet requires the strength of willpower capable of bending iron bars - ironically, the very lack of which may have already caused the weight problem. Another reason is our natural evolutionary safeguards that protect against times of famine. Eons-old emergency survival measures automatically kick in to preserve your unwanted wobbly bits when you consistently burn off more energy than you consume.

The Fat Fairy is not dissimilar to the Tooth Fairy, except instead of deposits of cash for teeth, the unfortunate recipient wakes up with unwanted lumps of body fat. According to some, these unwelcome visits often occur as the result of merely looking at a chocolate bar. Sadly, many people are not strangers to the Fat Fairy!

But possibly the most common reason of all is the necessity of breaking the habits that you've grown to love and cherish.

It's important to understand that habits are not just a mental issue, they're physical as well.

Humans, in general, are habitual creatures and there is some potent biochemistry going on in our body and brain that makes us cherish our habits – both good and bad. So, it's not just a case of breaking old habits, you've got to replace them with better ones - and learn to love them as well.

Without doubt, some dieters will succeed temporarily, dropping a dress size or two for a momentary period before it all piles back on again. Possibly, they've had partial success, getting halfway to their targets until suddenly, the siren call of the bacon sandwich or chocolate chip muffin becomes unbearable, and life resumes as before - albeit slightly lighter. For most, this will sound all too familiar.

So, the answer is not complicated: if you want to lose weight and feel good about yourself, you've got to make your new diet and lifestyle fit around you; around your way of thinking and on your terms, not the other way around, and we'll show you how.

Who are we to talk?

So, who are we to talk, and what gives us the authority to make these claims? Surely, we should boast a long string of important-looking letters after our names? At the very minimum we should be renowned for being the trainers on some reality-train-crash-weight-loss television show where we bully and beat the fat out of unfortunate, overweight contestants. Sorry, we cannot claim any of these accolades. The truth is we're just simple, ordinary folk, who now seem to be very successful at helping other simple, ordinary folk overcome their weight problems.

Between us we've about seventy years of accumulated nutritional knowledge and training experience.

We've had hundreds of thousands of hours honing our training skills in the gym, many tens of thousands of hours spent one-to-one with clients and countless hours of research and study.

Our classroom is the gym itself, face to face with people from every walk of life and to us that's a badge of honour we're proud to wear. Oddly enough however, it's safe to say that at times we've probably learned more from our clients than they did from us.

Every exercise programme we designed, and meal plan we created had to be redrawn each time for every new client: "You're having a laugh mate, I can't do that, I've got bad knees". Or, "Oh no, I can't eat that, it gives me terrible wind". Solving such mundane, yet typical problems such as dodgy joints and problematic bowels, along with clarifying misguided ideas about weight issues, diets and exercise is what we do best and led us to writing our books in the first place.

A little bit of common sense

Our solution to the problem is simple: we apply common sense. It's a philosophy we call **'weight-loss for grown-ups'**. We don't treat our clients as children, threatening them with the naughty step if they misbehave. We don't make them feel guilty when they slip-up - we're after consistency, not perfection. And we use our sense of humour, rather than cruelty or humiliation for motivation. For example, we would never tell anyone they are fat - or even overweight. Rather, we would suggest they are either under-height - or possibly the wrong species!*

---

* Well, Mr Smith, according to our charts, your weight would be ideal if you were eight feet tall, or a small hippo, perhaps. (We said it was our humour, we never said it was funny!)

But our driving principle is not to hold your hand because we believe that your issues are yours alone and only you can resolve them. It's vital that you learn to take responsibility for your life and take back control.

This is the presiding theme throughout this book and we'll slowly, bit by bit, show you how to do it.

What to expect

The book mirrors our usual approach to solving a client's weight problems. Therefore, it's based first and foremost on education. We work on the principle that if you give a man a fish, you feed him for a day; but teach him to fish and you feed him for life* *(14th century philosopher, Maimonides).*

Now, this book has nothing to do with fishing, but it is all about life, specifically, your life.

So, what can you expect from us?

Following a brief introduction to set the scene, it's straight into talking about food: helping you to decide what to eat and when to eat it. Then, we'll uncover the truth about what happens to your body when you lose weight and how to avoid the dreaded weight-loss plateau.

Following this, it's a quick dip into your mind, freeing you of the most common myths and misconceptions that regularly bewilder the unwary dieter. Finally, we'll tell you all about exercise and how to train smarter, not harder.

---

* It also gets him out of the house for the weekend, which is often a relief for his wife as well.

We believe that to win the weight-loss war you need to fully understand your opponent. Therefore, our aim is to provide you with both the necessary strategy and essential weaponry to claim complete victory.

Don't worry, it's not complicated (we're not clever enough for that).

You won't need a science degree; nor will you need to count calories, eat obscure vegetables or slurp vile tasting juices. You won't need to buy expensive kitchen gadgets, and exercise certainly won't involve a near-death-experience to see results. You may, however, need a tape measure and possibly an overdraft to fund the new wardrobe for when your old clothes no longer fit.

We're not promising that you can have all your cake and eat it, but you will get to enjoy the occasional slice.

So, enough waffle for now (there's plenty more to come), let's tell you a story about someone who's quick-fix diet made him as fat as a pig!

*****

Chapter 2:
As fat as a pig!

*'The quick-fix diet industry promises light at the end of the tunnel.
Unfortunately, it's that of an oncoming train: the 3.15 to Fatsville!'*
Paul & Ann

BECAUSE WE promote lifestyle change for weight loss it would be easy to assume that we are anti-diet. But we're not. Far from it in fact because we've spent years helping professional athletes become competition ready and this involves designing precise, calorie-controlled diets. Yet it's this experience that allows us to show that diets are not only unnecessary, but possibly the root cause of a person's weight problems. In fact, we recently came across a perfect illustration of the after effects of a badly designed, low-calorie diet.

We had a consultation with a potential male client who'd decided he wanted to get in fantastic shape. To give us an idea of what he wanted to look like he brought with him a photo of a friend, and a copy of the diet the friend had followed.

The guy in the image was in exceptionally good condition with a full six-pack on display (what we call in bodybuilding terminology, ripped or shredded). And his diet plan was a straight-forward, competitive bodybuilding plan: twelve weeks of extreme low-calories, lots of protein and about six to ten hours per week of hard training.

"Can you get me into the same condition?", he asked. "Yes", we said, "it can be done".

But we could see his face change when we explained some of the sacrifices that he would face. However, he thought he could manage it and said he wanted to think it over. Just before he left, I had a sudden thought: "Is this a recent photo?", I enquired. "No", he replied, "it's a couple of years old". "So, does your friend still look like this?" I asked. "Oh, no" the guy said without realising the irony of what he was about to say, "he's as fat as a pig now!". (Unfortunately, the guy never came back so we don't know if he ever tried it).

This is just one example out of hundreds that we've come across over the years. Incidentally, it's also why we're rarely impressed by the before and after photo. It's not to say that the 'after' photo doesn't deserve merit, because it certainly does. It's just we'd prefer to see the 'twelve-months-later' photo to see if the diet and training is still effective. And it's also why the only before and after photos you see on our website are of our professional body building clients. (And we only put them there just to show that it can be done – we respect out client's privacy too much to put their wobbly-bits on display just to promote our business.)

Whilst we have no scientific study to back us up, we would say that if you try too much, too soon, then you will regain all the weight, plus a further ten percent, in about half the time it took you to lose it.

Tip: When you see an impressive before and after photo advertising a diet or weight-loss product, just remember that the National Lottery only ever shows the one or two lucky jackpot winners, not the millions of losers.

The problem with diets

So, what's the problem with diets? Well, most diets suffer from three obstacles:

1. They are only a short-term solution to a long-term problem.
2. You can't live on a diet forever.
3. Diets require self-control. And, as we've already noted, the very lack of which may have created the situation.

However, we live in the real world and fully understand that some people will always feel the need to simply be told what to do: eat this, don't eat that; do this form of exercise, not that. (But it's not our preferred way of helping anyone to get in shape because we believe in teaching people how to do it for themselves.)

Although this may sound contradictory, we have no issue with any of our clients following the Paleo diet or joining weight-watchers, etc. Why? Because we're firm believers that if something works for you, no matter what we or anyone else says, then great. Our job is to offer guidance and support, not criticism.

Unfortunately, what most people don't understand is that all weight loss plans follow the same principles: reducing your calorie intake to less than your calorie expenditure. It's how they achieve this that raises our concerns. Nevertheless, there are some good diets on the market and some bad ones. There are not however, any perfect ones. All weight-loss plans, including ours, have pros and cons. The trick is find the ones that suit you as an individual.

So, what criteria do we use to determine a good diet?

What is a good diet?

Well, the underlying principle is simple:

- ✓ **You cannot measure the true success of any weight-loss plan in days, weeks, months, years or even in a decade, but in a lifetime. Because once the weight is off, it's got to stay off.**

Yes, you can lose weight for a holiday or a wedding but unless you fix the issues that caused the weight gain in the first place, it just comes back – often with a vengeance.

This is especially true if you lose the weight too quickly.

It's like borrowing money from a pay-day loan shark: the repayments are high, and the interest is extortionate. So, let's see how we put the above principle into action.

A good diet will:

- ✓ Teach you how to eat, not how to starve.
- ✓ Focus on fat loss and reducing inches rather than just losing weight.
- ✓ Promote lifestyle change, increased activity and healthy eating.
- ✓ Improve your relationship with food and not create an eating disorder.
- ✓ Provide a plan for long-term weight control.

On the flip-side, **it will not**:

- ✘ Permanently ban any food group.
- ✘ Use pseudo-science to establish its claims (e.g., chanting burns fat or carbs are calorie-free on weekdays when Leo is rising in Sagittarius).
- ✘ Have its own range of foods or arcane kitchen gadgets that you must buy.

Tip: It's important to realise that simply avoiding something only offers partial control. Yes, stopping having your chocolate digestives delivered by the pallet-load from Biscuits R'Us is a great start. But until you learn to eat just one or two - and not half the packet in one sitting - you haven't got full control of your diet. This is the reason why diets that ban certain foods or complete food groups eventually fail because they only reinforce the negative, i.e. the things you can't eat. **In fact, telling you that you can't have something often just increases your desire for it**.

Okay, let's get started with your diet.

*****

Chapter 3:
Food: The basics

'Excess fat is made from excess food and drink.
Now, what part of that did you not understand?'
Paul & Ann

THE FIRST consideration about designing any eating plan is that it's a totally subjective issue: it's relative to you and you only. It's not just personal likes and dislikes* but health, moral and religious considerations play a part as well. For example, you may be:

- ✓ A vegetarian who eats eggs and dairy but not meat or fish; or fish and dairy but not eggs and meat.
- ✓ Maybe you're completely vegan.
- ✓ You may have gone gluten free, sugar free, low fat, low sodium, no carb, non-dairy, soy-free, meat-free, wheat-free, paleo, macrobiotic, probiotic, antioxidant, non-GM, sustainable, raw, organic or local.
- ✓ Possibly your meat must be halal or kosher.
- ✓ You may even insist that your food must only be prepared by men or women who have never been intimate with their opposite sex (we've never really seen this one, but we bet it's out there somewhere).

---

* For example, Ann hates celery and fennel. I think parmesan cheese looks and smells like something scraped from a tramp's sock. So, the celery and parmesan cheese diet would be a definite no-no for us.

This alone makes it almost impossible to cover every variable, so we've decided to stick with the basic food groups - proteins, carbs and fats - and explain their role in planning a diet that will last you a lifetime.

The specifics: recipes, meal planners, detailed nutritional data, etc., are on our website where you can 'cherry-pick' the options that suit your own preferences. So, before we 'tuck in', let's have a quick chat about nutritious foods, filling in a food diary and reading food labels.

Nutritious food

This is a term that's bandied about so much, no one seems to wonder what it means anymore. We often hear, 'Ooo…, this is so nutritious; it's full of goodness'. But what exactly does it mean?

The word nutrition basically applies to the process of providing your body with the types of food necessary to support optimal health and growth. These foods come in two basic classifications:

1. **Macros**. These are nutrients we need in relatively large amounts (measured in grams): proteins, carbs, fats and water.
2. **Micros**. These are nutrients we need in tiny amounts (measured in milligrams or micrograms): vitamins, minerals, salt, electrolytes and phytonutrients (antioxidants), etc.

Generally-speaking, where the word nutritious is used, it usually refers to the micros. So, let's have a quick look at these tiny, but vital compounds.

Building your house

Humans require about forty essential micro-nutrients to function properly (in fact, we need hundreds more, but we can make them from the essential ones).

So, if we use an analogy of building a house, we could liken the macros to the building materials: bricks, cement, wood, etc. and micros to the builders of various trades: bricklayers, electricians, jointers, plumbers, etc.

Obviously, both materials and builders are essential for the job and a shortage of either leads to problems. So, when we talk about nutritious foods, we are really looking at foods that are full of essential builders.

Such as:

Vitamins & minerals

We'll discuss their role in detail in chapter 7

Salts & Electrolytes

These are minerals such as sodium or potassium and they are essential for every cell in your body to function properly. They are also responsible for maintaining blood pressure and fluid balance. Without sufficient salts and electrolytes, we would simply stop working.

Phytonutrients

These are plant-based chemical compounds that are thought to help prevent disease and promote a healthy immune system. Unlike vitamins, minerals, salts and electrolytes, they're not essential for life, but they may keep your body working properly. If we stretch our house-building analogy to breaking point, they would be the painters and decorators.

Empty calories

On the opposite side of nutritious, you may often come across the term 'empty calorie'. These are foods that will provide plenty of macros – usually in the form of simple sugars – but no micros. In fact, you could class empty calories as anti-nutrients because they do nothing but add extra work for your builders to deal with.

To summarise:

✓ A nutritious food is full of essential vitamins, minerals, salts, electrolytes and phytonutrients.

Tip: It's almost impossible to get every macro and micro in one food (potatoes come close). You really need a variety of foods from all the food groups to make sure you've have sufficient nutrition. Therefore, we never advocate completely removing any one foodstuff from your diet.

Are you a mindful or mindless eater?

Understanding the nutritional value of what passes your lips is the difference between being a mindful eater and a mindless one. Sadly, if you're the latter, you'll be forever getting unwelcome visits from the Fat Fairy.

So, you must, at the very least, start to read food labels. Also, keep some form of food diary for a while until you're more confident about what you're doing.

Now, we know food diaries are a pain in the bum and you want an easy life. One that doesn't involve anything mentally strenuous but trust us, you'll thank us for it at the end when the inches start to come off. Being mindful about your food is an essential part of a long-term, successful weight-loss plan and filling in a food diary will provide some vital data.

Such as:

✓ Often just writing down what you eat can make it instantly obvious what's going wrong.
✓ It will highlight eating patterns, cravings and habits, e.g., missing out meals or long gaps without food. It shows if you are binging on chocolate in the evening or always eating biscuits with tea or coffee in the afternoon.
✓ It provides a basic calorie value of your diet (and possibly the protein, carbs and fat content as well), which you can use as a benchmark.

Tip: If you don't want to fill in a food diary, just look in your cupboards or fridge – or at your shopping list – and see what you buy every week. Then, if you decide to make any changes to your diet, look to these foods first as they will usually account for the greatest number of calories consumed over the year.

In our other books and articles, we've talked about the elastic properties of calorie calculations (i.e., they can be out by up to 40%), but a food diary can be invaluable if you use the calorie values purely as a comparative tool to determine what's happening to your body. For example, is your weight currently stable or are you gaining or losing weight on your current calorie intake? Only when you've determined this relationship between what you're eating and what's happening, can you make the necessary changes to your food intake, e.g., cutting out sugar, becoming more active, etc.

You can use an online apps (we use MyFitnessPal, which has an option that allows us to see what our clients are eating as well) but we found that reading the food labels and writing it down is more educational and provides a deeper and more personal connection with your diet.

Tip: Some people do a food diary before they change their diet and lifestyle, others change first and use a food diary to keep track. It doesn't really matter how or what you do, so long as you do something to monitor your diet. Please understand that **if you don't know where you are now, you'll never be able to plan a route to where you want to be.**

Food rules

Okay, let's discuss a couple of basic food rules.

1. There is no such thing as a fattening food

It's important to stop categorising foods into fattening or diet options because you're missing a very important point.

Foods can be high calorie or low calorie, but you cannot classify any one, individual food as either 'fattening' or 'diet' because its energy value is relative to your lifestyle.

For example, **a cheeseburger is not fattening if you've just run a marathon!**

Equally, if you're about as energetic as a two-toed sloth having an afternoon nap, you could become obese from eating broccoli* if you ate enough of it. Not convinced? Well, look how fat cows get and they only eat grass!

So, stop thinking of 'fattening' and 'diet' foods and start thinking of your overall lifestyle, not just what you put in your mouth.

2. Mother nature knows best

Mother Nature provides very few high calorie meals. Now we realise that you may scoff at this statement but let us explain. If we were to put a bowl of sugar, a few egg yolks in a cup and a bowl of double cream in front of you and give you a spoon and tell you to dip in, you'd think we'd gone mad. Yet, if we did the same with a bowl of ice-cream, which is basically all three mixed together, you'd probably tuck in with unabandoned glee and end up licking the bowl clean.

Why we mention this is because nature never, ever provides a single food that is high in both fat and sugar. It's only when you start to mix the two that the calories pile up. Let's give you some examples:

(Note: the following covers most of the common foods that you will eat on a regular basis, so please read the relevant food labels for a more precise nutrient content.)

- ✓ All animal-based produce: chicken, fish, beef, etc., will be high in protein and virtually carb/sugar free. The fat content will vary

---

* (Interesting note: It would take 15kg of broccoli to supply enough calories to gain 1lb of fat. We wouldn't fancy being stuck in a lift with someone on the broccoli diet!)

depending upon which cut you use, how it's trimmed, and if you eat the skin or not (the skin often contains plenty of fat).

✓ Eggs are roughly equal amounts of protein and fat but are carb/sugar free.

✓ Meat substitutes, such as soya (Tofu), Quorn, etc., are high in protein, contain a small amount of carbs and very little fat.

✓ Fruits contain varying amounts of sugar but are low in protein and virtually fat free (an exception is an avocado).

✓ Any vegetable that you can eat, either raw or cooked from fresh on a hob (not a microwave), in less than ten minutes will be high in fibre, low in carbs/sugar and again, almost fat free. Protein content is usually low to moderate.

✓ Starchy carbs, such as potatoes, swede, etc., need a longer cooking time to break down insoluble fibre into edible starch. But again, they are relatively low in protein and contain almost no fat.

✓ Pulses: beans, chickpeas, lentils, etc., are slightly higher in protein than most veg, contain very little fat and are full of fibre. They are almost sugar-free and their carb content (starch) is low to moderate.

✓ In their natural, unrefined state, cereals such as oats, wheat, barley, rice, etc., are high in starchy carbs, low in sugar and fat, but have moderate amounts of protein.

✓ Nuts, seeds, avocados and coconuts are probably a few of the exceptions to the above because of their higher fat content. However, they are all low in simple sugars.

✓ Herbs and spices are virtually calorie free.

✓ The only unprocessed food that has roughly equal values of proteins, carbs and fat is fresh milk. But by volume, milk is mainly water and when processed into cheese or cream, most of the sugar is removed and you're left with a high fat, high protein food.

✓ Therefore, the best low-calorie food option is always Mother Nature.

There is a promising area of investigation into how the bacteria in your intestines may help you to optimise your weight-loss efforts. Apparently, your gut flora reacts positively to natural, unprocessed foods (Mother Nature again), especially fermented foods, such as sauerkraut, kimchi or miso.

It seems that these foods increase the healthy bacteria, which in turn, improves vital metabolic functions such as energy levels, mood and even sleep patterns. Because this research is in its infancy, we're not going into detail here (we don't want to cover a topic that may need amending at a later point). However, we're keeping a close eye on this exciting new research[*] and if you are interested, you can check out our website and keep up with the latest news.

Domestic science 101

We are carrying on with the theme of 'food rules' and now we're delving into a bit of domestic science. Why? Because quite frankly, we've come across so many people of the years who don't have the vaguest idea as to the nutritional content of their diet.

This doesn't entirely absolve anyone completely of blame as it's obvious that burgers, fries and fizzy drinks are all highly calorific and unhealthy. But then, did you know that the fat content in some tins of 'cream of' tomato/chicken/mushroom soup is nearly three times higher than a standard (54g) Mars Bar? It's not just things like soup either. Your 'healthy' chicken salad sandwich with a liberal spread of butter on the bread and a generous dollop of salad cream or mayonnaise will provide the same amount of fat as a 100g bar of milk chocolate and increase the calories to that of a Big Mac.

---

[*] On an interesting but unrelated note, it appears that bacteria are more intelligent than first thought. Apparently, when food is dropped on the floor, millions of hungry bacteria rush forwards but the king of the bacteria commands, 'Stop, you must wait five seconds, that is the law'. You learn something every day!

So, let's set the scene with a quick domestic science refresher course and begin by talking about the power of protein.

*****

Chapter 4:
Protein power

'Eggs are nutritious and great sources of protein -
unless they're preceded by the word Cadbury!'
Paul & Ann

PROTEIN IS probably the single most important nutrient in the body. The primary role of proteins is structural: they are the building blocks of your body. It's not just your muscle cells that are built from proteins, but your brain, bones, glands, skin, hair, etc., as well. In fact, very single cell in your body contains some form of essential protein. They also help to regulate your metabolism and act as a reserve energy source in times of famine (to your metabolism, prolonged, low-calorie diets are famines).

What foods contain protein?

Everything: if it's edible it contains protein. However, both content and quality will vary between proteins from the animal kingdom and the world of plants. For example, anything that was once a living, breathing creature will be high in protein, low in carbs and the fat content will vary depending upon which bits you eat. In contrast, plant-based foods: grains, pulses, veg and fruit will usually have more carbs than protein and are often almost fat-free. Pulses (beans, lentils, etc.) are also reliable sources of protein. Nuts are fine but are high in fat as well.

Tip: If you want to avoid animal foods, there are some great, high protein, meat-free substitutes: soya (tofu), Quorn and quinoa.

Benefits of a higher protein diet

There are some definite benefits to increasing your protein intake when you are trying to lose weight

- ✓ Helps prevent breakdown of muscle tissue to energy.
- ✓ Protein is more filling that carbs or fat and takes longer to digest. Therefore, it keeps the hunger pangs at bay.
- ✓ Your body uses energy to digest and metabolise everything you eat and drink. Now, anything that increases energy expenditure also causes an increase in your metabolic rate (a process called the Thermic Effect of Food). It's a bit like a bank taking a fee every time you move money across accounts. Your metabolism 'spends' about 25-30k/cals of energy to metabolise every 100k/cals of protein, whereas sugar and fat is only about 3-5k/cals per 100.
- ✓ Prolonged, low-calorie diets are known to create a fall in metabolic rate of up to 40%. Yet, a higher protein diet appears to prevent this. A recent study[1] showed that 20 obese patients followed a high protein yet low-calorie diet and lost an average of 20kg over a four-month period. But importantly, only had a 'statistically insignificant' drop in normal metabolic rate. This effect was attributed to the higher protein in the diet.

So, it doesn't take a genius to realise eating more protein is very beneficial when dieting.

We're not talking about binge-eating chicken by the bucket and drinking protein shakes like a steroid-fuelled body-builder, but just try to ensure at least two or three meals per day contains some quality protein.

Tip: Unless you have a family history of kidney stones or gout, or a doctor has told you otherwise, then adding a bit more protein to your diet should not cause any issues.

To give you an idea of the best protein options, that are also high in overall nutrition, we've put together a quick list.

Animal based proteins

Eggs

Eggs are probably the king of the complete protein, containing not only every amino-acid you need but lots of vitamins and minerals as well. A medium sized hen's egg has about 7 grams of protein and 6 grams of fat, with zero carbs.

Much of the bad press that eggs receive about causing high cholesterol is simply not true. Often, the studies - from which the scaremongering stories are based - are based on herbivore animals, such as rabbits and not omnivores like us. Animals that purely eat vegetables have no ability to metabolise any animal-based fats or cholesterol at all, whereas we can, so any results from these studies are irrelevant.

Obviously, if you're stuffing your face with burgers, chips, deep fried Mars bars and tons of other crappy foods, then eggs, especially fried, may contribute to your health problems. But if you eat a healthy, balanced diet, (along our guidelines), you would have to consume a massive amount of eggs to have a problem.

Tip: In the UK, the 'British Lion' symbol stamped on the egg will confirm the hens have been vaccinated against salmonella. Also, never buy cheap eggs from battery farmed hens. Apart from an utterly cruel and appalling way to treat a living creature, battery farming is such an intense procedure that the nutritional value of both the chicken and the egg will be severely reduced.

Finally, salmonella can live on the egg shell, so wash your hands after handling eggs.

Poultry (white meat)

Both chicken and turkey contain high amounts of protein with very little fat. Apart from some types of fish, they are the food of choice for a higher protein diet.

Like most animals, most of the fat is under the skin, so it's okay to cook with the skin on, but to keep the fat levels down, don't eat the skin. Another reason for not eating the skin is that if the animal has been exposed to any toxins, pollutants, pesticides, etc. they may be in the skin as well.

Again, like eggs, check the country of origin and it's worth noting that conscientious food retailers will advertise that their produce is 'morally farmed', meaning you're getting better treated and healthier animals.

Game birds & Duck

Game birds: Quail, Grouse, Pheasant and Duck, etc. are high in protein but usually higher in fat than chicken/turkey, especially duck, which is probably the fattiest of all birds. Unless you're a Lord of the Manor *(or a poacher)*, it's unlikely these meats will be a staple, regular protein source, so don't worry too much about an extra bit of fat. We would put game birds/duck in the same category as red meat (see overleaf) for consumption.

Seafood

Virtually any type of seafood you could eat will be high in protein, contains almost no carbs and most have very little fat as well (and what fat they do have is very, very healthy).

Seafood comes in two broad categories: fish and shellfish (crustaceans).

Fish

Some fish are higher in natural fats than others and whilst we recommend you try to include fish of any type in your diet, don't have 'fatty' fish more than three times per week (see below).

Unfortunately, whilst fish fats and oils are healthy, they may also contain tiny quantities of the pollutants and heavy metals that would be found in the fishing grounds and subsequently absorbed into the fat cells of the fish.

This concern also extends to 'farmed fish', (as opposed to fish that's been caught in its natural environment) but the health-related benefits of consuming fish oils far outweigh any slight potential detriment of avoiding them. Again, it may be worth doing your own research about this topic but it's always worth checking the label for origin - or asking the fishmonger if one is available - as it's in the interest of the food retailers to promote quality food.

- ✓ **Fatty fish**: Anchovies, Herrings, Kippers, Mackerel, Salmon, Sardines, Swordfish
- ✓ **Low-fat fish**: Bass, Bream, Cod, Flounder, Haddock, Hake, Halibut, Monkfish, Trout, Tuna.

Shellfish

Virtually all the shellfish you could eat are very low in both fat and carbs. In fact, some of them are so low in calories they are little more than water. The main problem with shellfish is that we rarely eat them in their natural state and are usually 'dressed' or put in a rich sauce. For example, a king-prawn has about ten calories, but a prawn cocktail will get close to two hundred, so watch out for the dressing and sauces.

As this chapter is all about protein, we've listed the high protein shellfish separately.

- ✓ **High protein shellfish**: Crab, Crayfish, Lobster
- ✓ **Low protein shellfish**: Mussels, Oysters, Prawns (shrimp), Scallops

Livestock (red meat)

Livestock are classified as cows (beef), pigs (pork) deer (venison) and sheep (lamb). Whilst all the meat from these animals will be high in protein and low in carbs, they can also be high in fat as well.

The amount of fat per serving will depend upon where on the animal the meat is taken from (the 'cut') and how much fat you trim off before eating.

Bear in mind though, that only the lean, choice cuts of meat get to the butchers, with the remaining lower quality, 'fattier' and cheaper cuts sold to be processed into burgers, sausages, sliced meat for sandwiches, etc. So, don't expect the best cuts of meat in your microwave lasagne.

From a health point of view, diets high in red meat consumption have been linked to serious illnesses, such as cancer, so again, try not to eat too often. During the week, we get our main protein intake from eggs, fish and chicken and save red meat for the weekend.

Dairy Products

Although cow's milk can cause digestive problems for some, most people in the western world will tolerate dairy pretty well. All dairy products are a good source of both protein (all amino-acids) and essential vitamins and minerals, but once processed, dairy produce can become very high in fat.

Whole milk contains roughly equal amounts of protein, carbs and fat; semi-skimmed has had most of the fat removed and skimmed is virtually fat free.

By volume, milk is mainly water but once churned into butter and cream or made into cheese, the water is reduced and the ratio of fat to protein and carbs rises dramatically. If you are thinking about increasing your protein intake by eating more cheese or lathering more butter on you toast, then don't!

Meat-free proteins

Of course, you don't just have to eat meat or fish to increase your protein intake because there are plenty of excellent vegetarian options. Probably the best one is Soya.

Soya Beans

All types of beans are good sources of protein - as well as fibre and vitamins and minerals - but soya beans not only have more protein than any other type of bean, they also have a complete range of amino-acids.

The 'soya' industry is now massive, as the bean is capable of being converted into a multitude of forms - dairy-type products, meat-substitute (Tofu), vegetable oil, sauces, etc. and they are all healthy, nutritious and low-fat.

Soya has been shown to help lower cholesterol, reduce the risk of colon cancer and is rich in phytoestrogens (which can reduce excess oestrogen production in women). All in all, it's an excellent meat replacement but there is a slight blip on the horizon. Because of high global demand for soya, scientists are genetically modifying (GM) soya to increase growth rates, crop yields, resistance to fungus and other pests, etc.

There are quite a few different GM versions on the market and the Food and Agriculture Industry, as well as the World Health Organisation feel they are perfectly safe.

However, there is some growing concern over the long-term effects of any plant that has had its genes altered. It should clearly state on the packaging whether the soya has been sourced from genetically modified crops or is GM free.

There is also some evidence that a high soya-based diet may lower testosterone production in men. But we think this is possibly a bit of 'scaremongering' by sections of the food industry that have vested interests in meat consumption (it's probably worth doing some research for yourself if you decide to make soya your principle source of protein).

Quorn

Quorn is classified as a 'mycoprotein' that has been grown in a fermentation vat. By feeding a form of fungus with sugar, vitamins, minerals and oxygen, a mycoprotein is produced, which, once dried, is then mixed with egg albumin (egg whites) to create a mince-like product. This is then shaped and flavoured for use in a wide variety of products, from burgers to pies and lasagnes.

It is relatively high in protein (although not quite as high as soya) and contains a full complement of amino-acids (possibly due to the added egg whites).

In its basic form, it's full of fibre and low in fat and the consensus of people who've tried it, is that it's a good meat substitute, although a small number of people (1 in 140,00) may have tolerance issues with mycoproteins. After changing production to include free range only eggs, the Vegetarian Society gave it its seal of approval.

Quinoa (pronounced Keen-wah)

Quinoa is a grain-like crop from which its seeds can be harvested and cooked like rice or processed into breakfast cereals and other foodstuffs. Again, it's relatively high in protein, (like Quorn) with a complete range of amino-acids.

It's low in fat and contains a decent range of vitamins and minerals. Apart from rinsing thoroughly - otherwise it's very bitter and acts as a laxative - it's another good food to consider if you decide to increase your protein intake without eating meat.

Beans (pulses & legumes)

Technically, the term 'bean' is specifically for the seeds of the broad or fava bean plant, although it's now commonly used to cover a wide range of vegetables (many of which are not actually beans). However, for the purposes of this chapter, anything with the word 'bean' attached to it will contain a decent amount of protein (but lacking a few essential amino-acids), as well as low in fat and packed with fibre, vitamins and minerals.

A definite must for anyone, regardless of its protein content or not (but don't blame us if you become a bit unpopular with friends and colleagues due to an increase of 'bottom burps' that accompanies a bean-rich diet).

Protein Supplements

The protein supplement industry is huge. It's no longer just powders anymore, there are protein bars, ready-made drinks, high protein yoghurts, bread and we've even seen high protein crisps. However, our advice with protein supplements is simple: they are a last resort only. Look to Mother Nature first for more protein and if you need more, then look at some supplement options (we've a lot more info about supplements on our website).

Quick guide to your top proteins

Okay, let's have a quick summary of your best protein options and we'll explain how to gauge your protein intake in chapter 9, when we talk about serving sizes

Top Ten Protein foods

1. Egg whites
2. Milk: cow, goat or soya are all good options
3. Soya products: Tofu, etc.
4. Poultry: chicken and turkey
5. Fish: especially oily fish such as salmon, mackerel and sardines
6. Livestock: beef, venison, pork
7. Quorn & Quinoa
8. Beans: any variety
9. Nuts: any type except peanuts
10. Protein supplements. Protein powders are often excellent but because they're supplements, we've put them last.

Okay, enough about protein, let's move on and talk about why you need to control your carbs

*****

Chapter 5:
Control your carbs

'Low carb diets are nothing new. In fact, they were popular in Ireland in the18th century; only then it was called the Potato Famine!'

Paul & Ann

POPULAR DIET trends in the late 1980s and early 90s all vilified fats as being the primary cause of the burgeoning obesity epidemic - the plague of fatness that had suddenly beset the western world. The clarion call was clear: 'Put down the lard and pick up a Pepsi!'. Whilst fats do play a major part in weight problems, they are not the only villain of the piece.

Now, if we were cynical people (we are - cynicism is genetic in South Yorkshire) we would look closely at the role of the sugar industry, for not only starting but perpetuating the myth that only fats are fattening. Why would we think this? Well, fats create what is called 'mouth-feel': that lovely soft, sensuous, moist taste and texture. It's something that we love because evolution has taught us over millions of years that fat is essential for life. It's not only high in calories but naturally occurring fats are packed with vital nutrients.

The great con-trick the sugar-based food industry has pulled is convincing you that products such as ice-cream, chocolate, etc. are 'fattening' due solely to their fat content, whereas the truth is the sugar is probably doing as much, if not more damage than the fat. (Note: The word 'fattening' is in inverted commas. Remember, there is no such thing as a fattening food, only a fattening diet.)

Okay, we'll stop here before this turns into a major rant about the multi-billion-dollar sugar industry and return to the subject of carb control.

What are carbs?

We can put carbohydrates into four broad categories

1. **Sugars**
2. **Starches**
3. **Soluble Fibre**
4. **Non-soluble Fibre**

There are a few others, such as alcohol, which we'll discuss in Chapter 16, but for simplicities sake, we'll stick to the above four categories.

Sugars are the simplest units of carbs; if sugar was compared to money, it would be a penny - the smallest coin of any currency. The main thing to remember about sugar is that it's the only type of carbohydrate that can be absorbed into the bloodstream. So, all forms of starch must convert (during the digestive process) to sugar prior to absorption. How does this work?

Imagine that you're at a Fun Fair and you need money to play the penny- slot machines. These machines will only accept pennies, so if you've got a 50p or £1 coin, it won't work - it must be broken down into pennies before you can play. Fortunately, the machines have a built-in cash dispenser that will eventually change any coin into the equivalent number of pennies.

However, anything above a 10p coin must be changed into smaller denominations first before it can be changed into pennies. For example, a £1 coin becomes two 50p pieces; each 50p piece becomes five 10p pieces and then each 10p coin becomes ten single pennies and you've finally ended up with a £1 coin converted into one hundred pennies.

This breakdown of large denominations into smaller currency is exactly what happens during digestion. **Starches** are the currency equivalent of one-pound coins and fifty-pence pieces.

Which is why starches take longer to digest than sugars, they must be broken down into ever decreasing smaller units before they can be absorbed.

But what about **soluble and non-soluble fibre** - what denomination are they?

If we push this sugar/currency analogy to breaking point, dietary fibre would be notes rather than coins. Unfortunately, our (cash dispensing) digestive system only changes coins and won't accept notes, so whilst soluble and non-soluble fibres have a massive nutritional value, they are not legal tender to our digestive system[*].

Okay, enough with the analogies, what do I do about eating carbs?

---

[*] *We were originally going to compare fibre to a Scottish £10 note. Whilst it's perfectly legal tender in the UK, no one south of the Scottish border ever believes this. Immediately they get one, they try to pass it on to someone else out of fear that it will be refused in the supermarket when it's the last tenner they've got in their purse or wallet. This would cleverly describe something that just 'passes through' the system but we thought it was an analogical-stretch too far!*

The contentious carbohydrate

The role of carbs in relation to weight management is still very debatable. Medical and scientific opinions vary between claims that sugar is the sole cause of the current obesity crisis to counterclaims that carbs, in general, have nothing to do with at all and weight issues are purely down to idleness and poor food choices.

To us (mere ordinary folk) the answer to the 'should we/shouldn't we eat carbs?' conundrum is a complete no-brainer: **excessive consumption of carbs, especially simple sugars, will make you fat and ruin your health**.

How do we know this?

Well, we don't have the luxury of sitting in 'lofty towers', pouring over databases and compiling statistics to come to our conclusions. We are the front line - we deliver the goods.

We are the ones advising our 'everyday–person-in-the–street' client how to effectively reduce their body fat.

And without exception, reducing their intake of simple, processed and refined sugars works! It's arguable whether this is due to an improvement in any specific metabolic and hormonal processes or simply the fact that they've reduced their calorie intake. Regardless - it still works!

Zero and low-carb diets are still popular, and again, our take on them is straight forward: humans evolved on natural carbs: fruit, nuts, root vegetables and berries. We would also argue that grains play a vital role in a healthy diet, despite what the anti-wheat fascists claim. And sorry Paleo-lovers, humans have been eating grains for tens of thousands of years.

In their unprocessed state, natural grains are packed with nutrition and fibre, helping to reduce cholesterol and improve insulin sensitivity, etc. However, we didn't evolve on refined and processed sugars: white bread, pastries, sweets, alcohol, chocolate, etc. So, whilst very nice, these foods are classed as 'empty calories' and not only will they affect your health, they're often the main culprits of a fattening diet!

Note: Insulin sensitivity occurs through prolonged consumption of high sugar foods and low levels of activity. The storage sites in the liver and muscles become 'insensitive' (they don't want the sugar) but the fat cells, usually in the liver and stomach, become more sensitive (they love the sugar). Insulin sensitivity is the precursor of type 2 diabetes. It's easily fixed by reducing sugar intake and increasing activity. We'll come back to this later.

So, to try and make some sense of which carbs will help and which will hinder your goals, we're going to offer a quick-guide to the contentious carbohydrate, and how, if you're not careful, it can cause metabolic mayhem.

So, let's have a quick summary of how carbs affect your body.

- ✓ The primary role of carbs in human metabolism is fuel. Therefore, if you are not active, you don't need them in large quantities.
- ✓ Try to ensure that most of your carb-based intake is from Mother Nature, i.e., it's unprocessed. This is primarily fruit and veg.
- ✓ Cooking – boiling, steaming, microwave, etc. - is a process that breaks down indigestible fibres into starchy carbs. Therefore, the longer a vegetable takes to cook, then the higher the carb (starch) content. So, almost any vegetable that can be eaten raw or cooked in a few minutes will be low in carbs
- ✓ Keep the high-energy, starchy carbs: rice potatoes, pasta, etc. to a minimum. However, if you are involved in high levels of exercise, then starchy carbs are vital for energy. In this case, we recommend that you only eat these foods on a training day (preferably after your workout when your muscle cells are highly sensitive to carbs).
- ✓ All carbs, regardless of their original form, break down into a simple sugar called glucose and this is your body's preferred energy source. Your cells will burn fat quite nicely, but glucose is always the first choice.
- ✓ Your cells have both a limited handling and storage capacity for glucose, making them easy to overload. Even in as little one meal, excess carbs can 'overspill' into your fat cells (note: this is very much an over-simplification, but the general idea is apt).

- ✓ Your fat cells don't suffer from handling or storage problems as your body makes new ones to cope with demand. The only way to increase your carb storage capacity is to build more muscle, but you'd have to build a lot to make a noticeable difference.
- ✓ Apart from playing a prominent role in developing type 2 diabetes and a host of other metabolic problems, a diet high in simple, refined sugars: alcohol, sweets, pastries, chocolate, etc. impacts badly on gut health and is often the true cause of IBS symptoms, causing inflammation, bloating, cramps, constipation, etc.
- ✓ Proteins and fats are essential nutrients, i.e., you must have them in your diet. Yet, if you stop eating carbs your body simply goes into ketosis (see over page). The insoluble fibre found in vegetables and pulses is very important for a healthy gut. So, on this basis, you can argue that some carbs are essential.

Note: Ketosis is a biological state where, due to a complete lack of carbs in your diet, your body converts specific fat-based structures (triglycerides) into a sugar-substitute called a ketone. When in ketosis your metabolism also converts proteins into energy at a faster rate.

Incidentally, a by-product of ketosis is an elevated level of a waste product called urea in your urine, bloodstream and sweat. The side-effects are not damaging but may lead to quite a severe headache until your body adapts to the ketones (and you may possibly smell of cat's wee). It's worth noting however that some people thrive on a low or zero-carb diet, whilst others simply can't function at all.

We'll come back to carbs and ketosis later in chapter 15, when we explain how to safely speed up the weight loss. For now, however, it's time to explore the world of fabulous fats.

*****

Chapter 6:
Fabulous fats

'Losing fat implies you might find it again.   Instead, throw it
all away and refuse to take it back'
Paul & Ann

THE FIRST THING to consider about fat is that it's not just a fuel source - or the annoying wobbly bit that hangs over your belt! Fat also performs vital roles in many metabolic functions. Not least cell structure and integrity, but also, the production of good cholesterol (HDL), sex hormones, and an optimally performing immune system. So, don't think that just because fat has over twice the calorie value of carbs or protein, you should eat less of it. In fact, if you eat 'fabulous fats' as opposed to 'flabby' fats, you're far less likely to pile on the pounds.

So, how do you tell fab from flabby? Unfortunately, it's not easy. Of everything that you can eat, dietary fat is possibly the most misrepresented and misunderstood nutrient of all. Sadly, it's been the subject of God knows how many witch-hunts and bad press over the years. However, the tide of scientific opinion seems to be returning them to favour.

For years, science told us that polyunsaturated fat was on the side of the angels and saturated fat was the spawn of Satan. New research now thinks that there are some fallen angels out there and a bit of devil-worship is okay.

(Note: the only consistent factor regarding the role of fat in human metabolism is the speed and regularity of the publication of contradictory studies. If you want to keep abreast of the latest research, check out our website where we'll do our best to offer some straight-forward advice.)

So, without going into a massive, overly-scientific explanation of the pros and cons of the diverse types of fats: mono, poly, saturated, oleic or linoleic, etc., we'll keep it simple.

- ✓ The naturally occurring fats and oils found in nuts, seeds, olives, milk, grains, fish - and even some red meat in small amounts - are fabulous and you should always include them in your eating plan (Mother Nature again).
- ✓ A lack of these essential fats will send the words, 'panic there's a famine' to your brain and immediately it will start to lower your metabolic rate faster than Usain Bolt in the Olympic finals. Fab fats are full of vitamins, minerals and tons of other vital nutrients necessary to maintain a fully functioning metabolism at maximum levels.
- ✓ What you don't need however, are processed fats from pies, pastries, chocolate, cream sauces, cooking oils, etc. Be wary of concentrated, full fat dairy products as well, such as cream and butter - and don't overdo the cheese (we think full-fat milk is fine).

But what about low-fat foods?

'Low-fat' is not always the best option

Food manufacturers are not stupid. They know that due to the current obesity epidemic and the fact that, for example, around one in four people in the UK are on a diet, (other countries have similar figures) there is a massive market for 'low-fat' produce. A situation from which they intend to squeeze the unwary consumer for every penny.

Tip: The words **'reduced fat'** on a food label indicate that the product contains 25 percent less fat than the original version. This does not, necessarily, mean that the product is low in fat. A product can only be labelled **'low fat'** if it contains 3 grams or less of fat per 100g of food. A claim of **'fat free'** indicates there is less than 0.5g of fat per 100g of food.

Yet, it doesn't necessarily mean these foods are low in calories. Why?

Some (not all) companies can be very sneaky with their reduced or low-fat options by simply replacing some the good fats in food with a type of concentrated sugar-syrup substitute. In fact, a reduced fat food item may be unhealthier in some respects than the original version of the product. Because it's not uncommon for additional salt and sugar to be added to the reduced fat food to make up for the loss of flavour that often results from lowering the fat content. This is another reason why you really should read food labels and if you're not sure what to look for, check out the governments website for advice: www.gov.uk/food-labelling-and-packaging

(Note: we are currently in the process of designing a new website and some of the topics we will cover in greater detail are food labelling and manufacturers sneaky practices, etc.)

Because of these and other chemically modified, unnatural procedures that food makers apply to our food, we generally ignore the low/reduced-fat versions unless there's a big difference in the amounts of saturated fat.

If saturated fat levels are considerably lower in the low or reduced fat option than the normal one, then it may be worth considering. However, if both the low/reduced-fat and regular products have about the same amount of saturated fat, then all that's happened is the manufacturer has replaced 'good' fat with sugar-syrup to be able to sell the product as a low or reduced fat option.

Again, you also really must look closely at food labels for hidden dairy fat, as it's often very easy to overlook. In the introduction to this book we mentioned that there's less fat in a standard Mars Bar than most creamed soups.

The same rule applies to pasta sauces, curries, ready-made meals, etc. The rule is that if it tastes smooth and creamy then it's highly likely to be either full of fat or a sugar-syrup type replacement.

Tip: If you love cooking, especially baking, bear in mind that a standard 250g pack of butter will contain nearly 2,000 calories. A small tub of single cream has about 400 calories, with clotted cream coming in at a whopping 1,200.

We usually split up foods high in natural fat over the course of the week. For example, we try to avoid having an oily fish such as salmon for dinner, if we'd had eggs for breakfast and had been nibbling nuts all day; we'd only choose one or two on each day of the week.

So, what should you eat?

Top ten 'fab' fat foods

1. Egg yolks
2. Oily fish – salmon, mackerel, sardines and kippers
3. Avocados
4. Extra virgin olive oil
5. Flaxseed oil
6. Nuts and seeds – walnuts and almonds
7. Dairy produce – Greek yoghurt, cottage cheese
8. Dark chocolate
9. Coconut oil
10. Tofu

If you look back to our top-ten list of proteins, you'll immediately see an overlap of many options, such as eggs, fish, dairy, soya produce and nuts, so it makes sense to build a healthy diet plan around these foods. The fly in the fat-ointment is their calorie value because it's just over twice the amount of proteins and carbs at 9k/cals per gram as opposed to 4k/cals per gram for protein and carbs.

Tip: To keep your calorie intake down, avoid whenever possible eating meals that are high in both fat and starchy carbs. For example, don't add a rich, creamy sauce to pasta or pile a heap of cheese on a jacket potato. Most of our meals options are either protein and fat or protein and starchy carbs.

We're almost at the end of the domestic science lesson and now it's time to consider the virtues of vitamins, minerals and water.

*****

Chapter 7:
Vitamins, minerals & water

'An average human is about 60% water. Maybe you're not overweight,
just waterlogged!'
Anonymous

VITAMINS AND MINERALS are essential for a healthy life. Whilst they have no calorie value in themselves (we can't burn them for fuel), they act as a 'spark plug' to your body's metabolic engine - getting it going and then keeping it running smoothly and maintaining all its functions.

At the end of this chapter, we've included a basic list of the most common vitamins and minerals, along with their best food sources. But our main aim is to discuss the role of the numerous pills and potions that are pushed upon the unwary.

Currently, there is a massive division of opinion about the efficacy of these types of supplements. On one side is the 'pro-supplement lobby', with their 'take our pills or you will die a slow, painful, lingering death' rhetoric. On the other, the anti-supplement 'it's all smoke and mirrors and you're just another imbecile who's easily parted from your money' sermonisers!

For every 'clinical' study that claims taking a specific supplemental vitamin, mineral or herb is vital to combat the strains and stresses of life's ailments, we could find another half-a-dozen that show it has little or no effect.

Let's imagine, for example, that you're feeling a bit tired, a little weary and run down - under the weather, so to speak (your usual 'get-up-and-go' has gone back to bed for a lie-down!).

You're busy, stressed, your diet's not brilliant and maybe you're lacking in 'something'. You're not sure what this 'something' is, so you check out your symptoms online or in your local herbal shop's handy guide to vitamins & minerals handbook and see if there's anything that may help.

Immediately, you see it's down to a lack of Vitamin B, in particular B6 & B12 because they're vital for converting carbs into energy. No, hang on a minute, it's definitely a lack of iron - you're not producing enough red blood cells. Scratch that - it's your immune system, you're lacking Vitamin C and zinc and probably some Echinacea as well just to be on the safe side. Ah…now you've got it: you're low in magnesium and therefore not producing enough of your feel-good hormone serotonin - that's why you feel run down and depressed. Wait a minute, what's this? It says that calcium interferes with magnesium absorption, so maybe you should stop drinking calcium-rich milk.

This is precisely the reason this chapter is not going to offer a 'lack of' or 'necessary for', one-size-fits-all description of the vitamin, mineral or herbal remedy industry - it's just too vague. The world is full of hypochondriacs due to the ambiguous information found in books and on the internet and we don't want to add any more. Virtually every common ailment under the Sun could be attributed to a lack of any particular vitamin or mineral.

Mankind has prospered for millions of years without supplements. Pay more attention to your diet and if you read anything about deficiencies on vitamins and minerals, look to eating the required foods, rather than immediately buy a bottle of pills to solve your problems.

We've put a simple table on the page 49 to list some of the best, natural food options for each vitamin and mineral. We're not going to include the Recommended Daily Amounts (RDA) because they're not much more than a good guess and are subjective to your age, gender, activity levels (daily needs) etc.

Also, we've only included the major vitamins and minerals (if you're eating most of the foods listed, you'll be getting the rest anyway, so don't lose sleep over them).

Most breakfast cereals are fortified with added vitamins and minerals and if you ate a decent serving of natural porridge oats with full-fat milk, a sprinkling of ground nuts/seeds, cinnamon or honey, you'll have pretty much covered just about everything (whether it's sufficient for you daily needs depend upon your 'daily needs' but it's a very good start to the day).

Tip: If you stand in the fruit and veg aisle of your local supermarket, you will see a variety of colours and this is an important point to consider, as each 'colour' contains different vitamins and minerals. So, go for the 'rainbow effect' on your plate, e.g. as many colours as possible, which will ensure you're getting a good variety of all the major vitamins and minerals.

The table on the next page is by no means complete, as there are probably as many food options missing as we've listed, but it should give you an idea of what you should try and eat.

Vitamins & minerals table

Vitamin	Best option	Other good sources (not listed in order)
A	Sweet Potato	Carrots, spinach, beef liver, milk, fish, eggs.
B (whole range)	Yeast, chickpeas, whole-grains	Oats, peanut butter, spinach. Most veg contain one or more of the vitamin B range. Most breakfast cereals are fortified with added Vitamin B
C	Red bell peppers, kiwi fruit	Citrus fruits, broccoli, beef liver
D	Salmon, swordfish (or other fatty fish)	Fish oil supplements
E	Yeast, seeds - flax/linseed/sunflower	Oats, wholegrain products, almonds
K	Kale	Most dark, leafy vegetables
Minerals	Best option	Other good sources (not listed in order)
Calcium	Low-fat yoghurts	All dairy produce, any dark leafy vegetables, oats
Iron	Any red meat, fish or poultry, especially the liver	Beans, lentils, oats, dark leafy vegetables
Magnesium	Any wheat bran product	Almonds, cashews, most green vegetables
Potassium	Sweet potatoes	Bananas, tomatoes, red meat, poultry, oats
Zinc	Oysters, crab meat	Grains, nuts, seeds, eggs, red meat and poultry

Mega-dose myths

Much of the hype about the wonderful curative powers of mega-doses of vitamins and minerals are not available 'over the counter' because they are usually the result of being administered intravenously, (via injection or a 'drip') under medical supervision.

They also mislead by relating test results and studies that are not relevant to us. For example, it's claimed Vitamin C kills cancer cells. This, in fact, is true, if the cancer cells are in a petri dish under laboratory conditions. However, bleach and vinegar also kill cancer cells in a petri dish! Yet, we very much doubt your local doctor would give you a prescription for either of those!

Your intestinal tract is simply not capable of absorbing these massive doses, so apart from upsetting your stomach and potentially blocking the absorption of other nutrients, they end up in the toilet.

If you are taking mineral supplements, then unless they are in a 'chelated' form, they will not absorb very well. Again, to avoid over-complication, 'chelated'[2] basically means that they are in the same state as would be found in nature. This means that your intestines recognise them as a natural, organic compound (most minerals are inorganic metals), allowing them to pass through the intestinal wall into the bloodstream. Otherwise, once again, they end up down the loo.

Tip: If you're not sure about what you need, then arrange for a blood test at your local GP. They will be able to tell you if you are low in most vitamins or minerals, especially iron or vitamin D.

Wonderful water

Let's not forget about water. It goes without saying that you must drink sufficient fluids but the advice about two litres per day is again, rather vague.

You can tell if you're drinking enough fluid with a simple test.

First thing in the morning your pee looks concentrated and often has a distinct odour. By mid-day it should be a lot lighter and odourless, and by mid-afternoon it should be almost clear or the colour of pale straw. If it's not, then either your protein intake is too high or, more than likely, you're not drinking enough water. Conversely, if you're peeing every hour, you are drinking too much.

Tip: It's not true that tea and coffee are powerful diuretics. Yes, they may slightly increase your urine output but unless you are drinking a double espresso every five minutes, you will still retain most of the water from the drink.

Okay, the domestic science lesson is now over and it's time to have a look at what to eat. And for that, we're going to show you how to determine which foods are super, which are safe, which are sneaky, and which are downright scandalous.

*****

Chapter 8:
Super, safe and sneaky foods

'It's ironic that Homer Simpson, originally created as a parody of gluttony and sloth, now seems to be a role model'
Paul & Ann

THE PURPOSE of this book is to make your life as simple as possible. So, with that idea in mind, we've created four, general food categories that will help you to identify what you should be eating. We're going to look at some **super, safe, sneaky and scandalous** food options.

Note: It's important to apply a little bit of common sense to these categories because they're not written in stone. They're very general and far from complete, and they only cover the most popular, basic foods. The classifications apply to foods in their natural state without dressings, sauces or fillings. Also, any necessary cooking or preparation methods do not add further calories, e.g. frying or soaking in a marinade. Finally, the comparative cooking times for veg are based on boiling in water using a hob, not by microwave or a steam/pressure cooker.

We recommend that you only apply them to the foods that you would eat on a regular basis and don't worry too much about any 'sneaky foods' if you only eat them occasionally, e.g., on special occasions or a couple of times per month.

Super foods are the best

They're generally low-calorie and full of healthy nutrition. They should form the base from which you build your campaign to win the inch war. If it's in the super category, don't give it a second thought about eating it.

Safe foods are great

These will also be full of healthy nutrition, but their calorie values may be slightly higher or normal portion sizes bigger. So, to be on the safe side, you must be a little more cautious with your selections.

Sneaky foods are okay in moderation

Some sneaky foods are not what they seem. Whilst they are nutritious, they are higher in calories than you may think and will sneak up on your fat cells if you're not careful.

Scandalous foods are treats and special occasions

This would cover all the foods that you shouldn't be eating. However, the list would be longer than the entire book and it's likely that you already know what they are i.e., the ones that have already caused the weight problems!

To offer you an idea as to how these categories work, we've added a short list on the next few pages. We'll apply them again when we look at your meal options and you can find even more information on our website.

Note: Unless you are following of our calorie cycling plans (Chapter 15) don't worry unduly about the difference between most super and safe categories.

Animal based foods (meat, eggs, dairy)

Super

- ✓ Skinless chicken, turkey. All types of fish, including shellfish.
- ✓ Eggs: boiled, poached, omelette, scrambled. In fact, anyway you like except fried (they're Sneaky).
- ✓ Natural yoghurt including the pro-biotic and high-protein options. All unsweetened goat, sheep, soya, almond and coconut alternatives to dairy produce.

Safe

- ✓ Steak and lean cuts of beef, pork, gammon & ham. All game birds. Deli cuts (not reformed) of beef, pork, ham, etc. Lean minced steak.
- ✓ Cow's milk (all types). Cottage cheese.

Sneaky

- ✓ Lamb
- ✓ Fried eggs
- ✓ Quality burgers, sausages, etc
- ✓ Lean bacon
- ✓ All variations of hard/soft cheese and single/double cream. Halloumi.

Scandalous

- ✗ Reformed or 'formed from' packet meat
- ✗ Take away burgers, kebabs, etc.
- ✗ Cheap, minced beef

Plant-based foods
(meat substitutes, veg, fruit, grains, nuts, herbs & seeds)

Super

- ✓ All variations of tofu, tempeh, Seitan, Quorn, quinoa, mushroom, etc.
- ✓ Any veg that can be eaten raw, e.g., all salad veggies.
- ✓ Any veg that takes under 10mins to cook (on a hob): broccoli, cabbage, cauliflower, peas, carrots, etc.
- ✓ Garlic, kale, alfalfa, lentils, chick peas and any type of bean.
- ✓ Traditional porridge oats.
- ✓ All types of fruit - especially berries and avocados - but don't get excessive with bananas or grapes.
- ✓ Almonds, brazil nuts and walnuts.
- ✓ All seeds, herbs and spices.

Safe

- ✓ Rice, sweet potato (Yams), new potatoes, swede, turnip, parsnip, pasta (all varieties).
- ✓ Wraps, pitta, ciabatta, panini & artisan-style breads from a bakery (spelt, sourdough, etc.).
- ✓ Falafel, hummus. Olives (in moderation)
- ✓ Unsweetened cereals: Weetabix, Shreddies, muesli, granola, etc. (but beware of sugar content if they contain dried fruit).
- ✓ Cashews.

Sneaky

- ✓ Jacket potato. Any form of processed potato products: chips, waffles, etc. Commercially-made, sliced bread. Pre-packaged sandwiches, bagels. Danish pastries.
- ✓ Kiddies cereals and any cereal that can be eaten straight from the packet will be sweetened and high in sugar.
- ✓ All types of dried fruit. Honey
- ✓ Dry roasted peanuts. Peanut butter.

Scandalous

- ✗ Any deep-fried potato products
- ✗ Fruit juice (cheap concentrate)
- ✗ Tinned fruit in syrup

Fats, oils and sauces

Super

- ✓ Olive oil, coconut oil, flaxseed oil

Safe

- ✓ Rapeseed oil, sunflower oil

- ✓ Non-dairy butter substitutes (Bertolli, Pure, etc).
- ✓ Tomato and brown sauces
- ✓ All chutneys and pickles

Sneaky

- ✓ Any type of creamed sauce: hollandaise, tartar, béarnaise, etc.
- ✓ Creamy pasta/rice sauces
- ✓ Margarine

Scandalous

- ✗ Cheap vegetable/cooking oil
- ✗ Anything that has 'contains hydrogenated fat' on the food label.

Deserts and Snacks

Super

- ✓ Crisp breads (unsweetened)

Safe

- ✓ Tinned fruit in juice.
- ✓ Frozen yoghurt.
- ✓ Dark chocolate
- ✓ Rice cakes

Sneaky

- ✓ Cereal & granola bars

Scandalous

- ✗ Just about everything that's full of both sugar and fat: chocolate biscuits, cakes, ice cream, trifle, etc, etc.

Okay, let's put these foods into action and have a quick look at making the best choices for your super diet.

Chapter 9:
Your super diet

'A cake in each hand does not constitute a balanced diet!'
Paul & Ann

NOW, THIS is where we get to the tricky bit. Usually, when we design a meal plan for a client, we've already had a long chat about their goals. Plus, we'll have discussed their food preferences; we'll know how much they weigh and how active they are (or will be). Basically, we've got something to work from. Here, we're only guessing. So, we'll keep it simple and stay with a traditional western-style diet, a regular supermarket and assume that you don't have any allergies, intolerances or medical conditions that exclude certain foods (please see the disclaimer at the beginning of the book). We don't know if you have any moral or religious restrictions on your diet, so please use alternatives food options as you deem necessary.

Serving sizes

Before we get to the food, we'll have a quick word about gauging portion sizes. Now, our philosophy is to try and make your life as simple as possible, so we'll explain a couple of methods and you can decide which one suits you best.

1. Complicated: count calories and weigh food

If you like to be precise, then buy some accurate kitchen scales and use some form of calorie counting.

This could be a book or an online food database such as MyFitnessPal. We're not big lovers of using 'calories' to determine how much you should eat. In chapter 17, we'll offer a full explanation but suffice to say that slavishly counting calories is like measuring your waistline with an elastic tape measure. We not saying not to do it, just be aware that it's not accurate. Generally, we use calorie values as a comparison between similar foods, rather than following a daily amount.

2. Simple: use your hand as gauge for portion sizes

Whilst this is less accurate, it does have the great advantage of determining how much you should eat relative to your size. This is great when you have, for example, two people of different sizes eating similar plates of food.

How does this work?

- ✓ One portion of meat or fish (or meat substitute) should be about the same size and thickness as your hand.
- ✓ One portion of vegetables should fit into both hands cupped together.
- ✓ One portion of uncooked starchy carbs (potatoes, rice, pasta, etc.) should fit into one cupped hand. If you don't want to use a cupped hand, you could simply use a cup or a mug to gauge the amount (and use that same level, e.g., ½ or ¾ full as one portion).
- ✓ One portion of bread should be about the same size and thickness of your hand.
- ✓ One portion of butter/spread would be the same size as the top half of your thumb
- ✓ One portion of nuts would cover half the palm of your hand

The important thing to remember is that your results are more important than the methods used to gauge the quantity of foods in your diet. Only when you see the results will you know if you need to make any alterations to what you are eating.

Notes: We're going to talk about food options in general, we're not covering any recipes. At the end of each chapter, we'll add a few ideas under our super, safe, sneaky options. Sorry, we can't be more specific but there are simply too many foods on the market to offer a full listing (most online food databases now carry over 100,000 foods). If you're looking for some brilliant recipes, then check out BBC's good food guide (www.bbcgoodfood.com).

All the listings for breakfast, lunch, evening meal, snacks and desserts are interchangeable.

Okay, let's start with breakfast.

*****

Chapter 10:
Breakfast

'Start the day with determination. Finish it with satisfaction.'
Anonymous

THE FIRST THING to understand is that breakfast is not necessarily the most important meal of the day. In truth, it doesn't 'kick-start' your metabolism – well, no more than any other meal does. Any meal, at any time of day, causes an increase in your usual metabolic rate (a process called the Thermic Effect of Food). Which is often why you can feel warmer after a large meal: any increase in metabolism causes a rise in body temperature.

Unfortunately, an overnight fast is simply not long enough to create a noticeable drop in your usual metabolic rate. In fact, you'd need to starve for about five days at least for it to fall below normal levels. However, there's no doubt that breakfast-eaters are less likely to have the same weight problems as breakfast-skippers. Also, food first thing in the morning can help to reduce levels of a stress hormone called cortisol. It's also been shown to reduce afternoon cravings for sugary-foods and high-carb evening meals. But everything you eat has a calorie value and breakfast is no different – it all adds to the total.

Some people can't face food when they rise, others are starving. Bear in mind that we are creatures of habit and often we're not hungry first thing because we've got out of the habit of eating breakfast.

However, if you recognise yourself as chronically stressed, or you see from your food diary that you have an afternoon sugar craving, then it may be worth trying to start the day with something light.

Tip: Try some yoghurt and fruit, and maybe build it up to something more substantial as time progresses. You may soon find that you are hungry again at breakfast and may also have resolved your stress and cravings. Otherwise, we advise that you listen to your body and don't eat something that you don't want, just because the 'you-must-eat-breakfast-fascists' say so.

But what is the best thing to eat in the morning? Ideally, you would eat something that is healthy, nutritious, filling and doesn't cause a sugar-spike.

So, let's see what's on the 'super' breakfast menu.

Eggs

Possibly, the best breakfast food is an egg. You can have it any way you like: scrambled, boiled, poached, omelette, etc. but avoid eating fried eggs on a regular basis. Eggs are full of protein, healthy fats, vitamins, minerals and keep you full for ages. Egg whites are all protein and the yolks are mainly fat. However, the yolk is where most of the nutrition is, so don't just eat the white.

Traditional porridge oats

After eggs, porridge oats come in a close second. Again, packed to the hilt with nutrition as well as with cholesterol lowering properties. Traditional porridge oats are not only very filling, they cause fewer intolerance/bloating problems than most other breakfast cereals. You can find some great muesli/granola type cereals that consist mainly of oats, but they can also contain lots of hidden sugars in the added honey and/or dried fruit. So, look at the label if you're watching your sugar intake.

Also, you may find that oats from the two-minute microwave pots and sachets are not as filling. We cook traditional, rolled oats in a microwave and it only takes four to five minutes with a bit of stirring.

Tip: If you find porridge bland, add a teaspoon of vanilla essence, sprinkle cinnamon on top or add some berries. To increase your protein, cook it with a little bit less liquid than normal.

Then mix up a serving of protein powder (flavour of your choice) and stir in immediately after it's cooked (you may have to play around with the total amount of liquid depending upon how thick you like your porridge). This adds a bit more protein and provides some extra taste as well.

Other Cereals

Breakfast cereal makers are sneaky, latching onto every eating trend possible and if they can't find a good one, they'll make their own. They know that many people are in a rush in the morning and target them with clever adverts offering healthy and filling breakfasts in a biscuit, or even in a chocolate flavoured drink (hang your head in shame for this one, Weetabix).

Let's get one thing straight: claiming that you can have a 'healthy, chocolate' breakfast is complete nonsense. It's like saying that smoking is good for you because the tar from the cigarettes provides a protective coating on the lungs! Also, despite what the adverts claim, a breakfast biscuit is just a biscuit - only about five times more expensive!

Still not sure?

Imagine that you've just sat down to a so-called 'healthy' breakfast of a bowl of 'wholegrain choc-a-bix-wheat-a-hoops', (catchy title, don't you think?) with semi-skimmed milk and a glass of orange juice. First, if you eat the recommended serving size, you'll just about manage a mouthful before it's all gone. Therefore, if you're a normal adult, your serving size will be about three times bigger than the amount on the packet.

Now, you may not realise it but with the added sugar in the cereal, as well as the sugar in the juice and milk, you're about to eat the equivalent of a dozen teaspoons-worth (about 60-70g) of sugar! Just try putting that amount in your tea or coffee and see what it tastes like.

And if little Timmy or Suzie eats a similar breakfast, is there any wonder why they're bouncing off the walls all morning and then can't keep awake in the afternoon? Maybe it's not ADHD after all!

Tip: All natural, unprocessed cereals - from oats to wheat, rice and pasta, etc., have all the taste and texture of cardboard. So, to make them palatable sugar is added! It's easy to test: if you could eat the cereal straight from the pack and it tastes nice, it's been heavily sweetened. Therefore, avoid it like the plague if you can. Other than oats, the only cereals that we would recommend eating for breakfast - on a regular basis - are Weetabix or Shredded Wheat (or their generic supermarket versions). Why? Because if you tried to eat them without milk you'll instantly see what we mean - the box would be tastier!

Fruit and Yoghurt

If you're not much of a breakfast person, just take some fresh fruit/berries and pour on some natural yoghurt. This is our favourite breakfast in the summer months (usually about three days in this bloody country!). It's light, quick and easy to prepare. Fresh fruit/berries are lower in sugar than dried fruit and natural yoghurt is high in probiotics, which may improve gut health. If you don't tolerate dairy, there are some great alternatives in soya, sheep or goat's milk.

Tip: If you prefer it a little more filling (and with extra protein), try a version of yoghurt called Quark. Also, Scandinavian food company, Arla make some great high protein yoghurts but just beware of the sugar content in some of the flavoured versions. Finally, we don't bother with low-fat, or fat-free yoghurts because firstly, most of the good nutrition is in the fat. And secondly, the missing fat is often replaced with a gelatinous substance called Modified Maize Starch (MMS is also known as wallpaper paste). To us, this outweighs the slightly higher calorie value.

Toast

A couple of slices of toast, liberally covered with jam, marmalade or some other spread must be the most common breakfast in the UK. But hang on a moment, isn't bread evil?

According to some, eating bread will not only make you fat, it'll give you dementia, cause your hair to fall out and is possibly entirely to blame for the current Middle Eastern crisis! When we tell our clients that we eat bread, they often look at us as if we'd just said we used to be pen-pals with Saddam Hussein.

A word about bread

There's a lot written about bread these days: intolerances, bloating, IBS, etc., and sadly much of it is true - particularly in the case of commercially made, sliced bread. Many of the cereal crops used to make flour for bread, such as wheat, barley, rye, oats and spelt, contain an almost indigestible protein called gluten. Making bread involves a lengthy kneading process to make the gluten absorb water and become more elastic, allowing the baker to shape the bread. The mixture also needs time (anything from 30 minutes to a few hours) to 'prove'. This process allows all the necessary chemical reactions between the flour, yeast and oxygen to take place, ultimately creating the 'doughy', soft taste when baked. Unfortunately, the gluten dries out quite easily once cooked and the bread quickly starts to go stale.

Commercial baking processes change this. To increase productivity - and thereby reduce costs - various additives are necessary to both speed up the rate at which the bread would normally prove. It also stops the gluten from drying out, prolonging the shelf-life of the bread. We feel that in many cases, it's these additives and alterations to the natural baking processes that causes the problems, rather than bread itself.

Unfortunately, once you develop a problem with gluten intolerance it's difficult to overcome because gluten is everywhere.

It's found in dozens of other products from pizzas to pies and ketchup to ice-cream. Its natural elastic properties make it another ideal filler for low-fat products and ready-made, microwavable meals. (Note: you can buy gluten-free bread, but it may often be higher in calories than normal due to the added sugar necessary to maintain its texture).

Most cheap white bread is made from highly processed flour that has had all the fibre and nutrition removed, so it's basically just compressed sugar. Wholemeal/wholegrain bread, whilst much healthier (full of fibre and vitamins), also struggles to stay moist and often contains extra salt to stop it going dry. Bread, by itself, is not necessarily calorific (about 90k/cals per slice) but when you slather it with butter and jam or marmalade, you can easily double its calorie value. The 'sugar spike' received from cheap forms of white toast may leave you craving for the biscuit tin by 10am. Generally-speaking, artisan or bakery-made bread is what we class as a 'safe' option and sliced bread is out and out sneaky.

Tip: Bread is such a staple part of our daily diet it's difficult to replace. However, we have yet to come across anyone who has not felt better for either cutting out or reducing their intake of popular-branded sliced bread. If you must have bread, try breads such as sourdough, ciabatta, Panini and focaccia. Flat breads like pitta are possibly healthier alternatives as they are made with olive oil, have less yeast or other chemicals and are usually meant to be eaten on the day of baking (but they can be quite high calorie). We've also found tortilla wraps to be good replacements for bread, as well as rice cakes and crisp-breads, such as Ryvita.

What's left for breakfast?

Walk down the breakfast food aisles of your local supermarket and you are bombarded with options, many of which claim to be healthy and wholesome but try to pick carefully. It may be making such claims because it's made with oats or whole grains, but it could be full of added sugar.

Be wary of anything that has more than 12-15g of sugar per dry serving (or 20g including milk).

Remember, there is no such thing as a fattening food, only a fattening diet, so keep the bacon/sausage sarnies, buttered croissants, crumpets, muffins, doughnuts, etc. to a minimum.

Right, let's have a shopping list for breakfast.

Super

- ✓ Eggs: boiled, poached, omelette
- ✓ Porridge oats: traditional
- ✓ Natural yoghurt & berries
- ✓ Salmon & avocado on crispbreads/toast
- ✓ Mackerel, kippers, etc.
- ✓ Weetabix, shreddies, wholegrain bran
- ✓ Vegetarian options using Tofu, Quorn, etc.
- ✓ Add any fresh fruit, nuts and seeds to the above
- ✓ Milk: semi-skimmed cow's or goat's. Unsweetened almond, coconut, soya & rice milk (if you are just adding milk to cereal, then don't worry if it's full fat or sweetened).

Safe

- ✓ Eggs: fried (not too often)
- ✓ Porridge oats: microwave or Ready Brek
- ✓ Toast: bakery made sourdough or ciabatta
- ✓ Peanut butter (not applied with a trowel!)
- ✓ Muesli & Granola (but be aware of sugar content)
- ✓ Protein shakes/smoothies you've made yourself
- ✓ Full-fat cow's milk (essential for children)

Sneaky

- ✓ Eggs: hollandaise, benedict, etc.
- ✓ Toast: commercially made, sliced
- ✓ Kiddies breakfast cereals
- ✓ Breakfast biscuits, cereal & protein bars
- ✓ Peanut butter. Honey.
- ✓ All types of commercially-made smoothies, fruit juice and dried fruit

Scandalous

- ✗ Full English

- ✗ Sausage and bacon sandwiches
- ✗ Danish pasties: croissants, etc.
- ✗ Any cereal that contains chocolate
- ✗ Coffee with hidden high sugar/cream content

Super Breakfast Plan

(All values are approximate, please check relevant food labels.)

BREAKFAST	Protein	Carbs	Fat	Cals
Breakfast cereal: 50g or ½ cup: Weetabix/Shredded Wheat/Bran/Porridge, etc. With s/skim milk	7g	30g	3g	175
Egg: poached or boiled	7g	trace	6g	82
Eggs x 2 - scrambled	13g	1g	14g	182
Toast x 1 slice buttered with peanut butter	4g 4g	15g 25g	6g 6g	130 170
Mackerel: tinned with tomato sauce	14g	2g	11g	163
Crisp bread x 1 (dry)	1g	6g	0.5g	33
Salmon flakes: 50g ½ avocado	11g 2g	4g 6g	6g 12g	118 140
Fruit: 1 x apple, pear, orange, etc. -banana - berries (average) -	1g 1g 1g	11g 25g 14g	0g 0g 0g	48 104 60
Yoghurt: 125g (½ cup) Natural (full fat) - Greek (full fat) - Flavoured (Low-fat)	7g 8g 5g	10g 3g 22g	4g 13g 1g	104 161 117

*****

Chapter 11:
Lunch

'Junk food only satisfies your stomach. Looking good satisfies your life'
Anonymous

A GOOD LUNCH can be slightly more problematic than breakfast or dinner. On one hand, we advise clients to try and eat their carbs during the day when they're generally more active (you don't need a lot of energy to sit on your bum and watch Telly). Yet, on the other hand, a high carb lunch can leave you feeling lethargic and sleepy in the afternoon.

Humans naturally have a dip in energy levels about 2pm and if you add in a sizable lunch that diverts blood from the brain to the stomach for digestion, you'll end up needing to snort caffeine just to stay awake! Obviously, not everyone suffers with this but there's tons of evidence[3] that suggests it's a widespread problem.

Tip: Eat a little less at breakfast and lunch, and slightly more at your morning and mid-afternoon breaks to balance your food out for the day. This has the added benefit of not feeling starving when lunch and dinner come along, and you won't overeat as much.

So, let's look at a few options.

Salad box

Possibly the best lunch is one you've made yourself. Use fresh salad vegetables such as assorted spinach/rocket/herb leaves, tomatoes, bell peppers, etc. as a nutritious, low-calorie base.

Then, add either diced chicken, salmon, tuna or a chopped up boiled egg for some protein. If you want some carbs, throw in a small handful of pasta or new potatoes, or a handful of pre-cooked kidney/haricot beans. Finally, drizzle on some balsamic vinegar, olive oil or light salad dressing and you have a fantastic, low-calorie/low-carb, fully balanced lunch.

Sandwiches

The humble sandwich is probably the most common lunch in the Western world. The permutations for a good sandwich are almost endless. However, rather than buy one from a shop, try to make you own. You're more in control of the ingredients, especially the sneaky, hidden calories such as butter (or margarine), salad cream, mayonnaise, etc.

Tip: Try wraps instead of bread. Calorie-wise, a wrap will be just about equal to a couple of slices of bread (or a bread cake, bap, roll, etc.) but wraps are never buttered. Nor do they contain anywhere near the amount of yeast or chemical improvers that bread does. Most of our clients have found that changing from bread to wraps is far easier on their stomach.

A Light Lunch

If you don't want too much at lunch, then crisp breads or rice cakes, etc. are a great alternative to sandwiches. There's an almost infinite range of toppings but our favourite is any variety of cottage cheese - natural, pineapple, chives, etc. Cottage cheese takes ages to digest and contains an amino-acid called Tryptophan - essential to produce serotonin, your 'feel good' hormone. For this reason, cottage cheese is also a great pre-bedtime snack.

Something hot?

If you want something either warmer or more filling for lunch, then look at chilli and rice, tuna and pasta or a jacket potato with baked beans. It's likely that your calorie intake won't be much higher than 5ook/cals - about the same as a pre-packaged sandwich from the garage.

The trick to keep your calories down is to make sure that if you are having a high-carb lunch, don't mix it with a high-fat food. For example, don't pile butter and cheese onto the potato or use a creamy sauce for the pasta. Soup is another option but watch out for the fat content of 'cream of' soups and obviously, watch the bread (try crispbreads instead).

Okay, let's have a shopping list for lunch.

Super

✓ All salad/raw vegetables
✓ Fillings for sandwiches/wraps/pasta/potatoes, etc: lean cuts of chicken breast, turkey, beef and pork. Tuna, salmon, baked beans, lean chilli.
✓ Crispbreads & Rice cakes
✓ Cottage cheese

Safe

✓ Wraps & ciabatta bread. Traditionally baked sourdough bread.
✓ New potatoes, rice, couscous and pasta (only one portion: 1 x cupped hand)
✓ Jacket potato (small to medium, without butter)
✓ Hummus & falafel

Sneaky

✓ Commercially made, sliced-bread. Bagels
✓ Most cheeses, especially cream cheese
✓ 'Cream of' of soups
✓ Packet, sliced meat (reformed wafer-thin ham, beef, etc)

Scandalous

✗ Pre-packaged sandwiches and wraps (it's not just the calories but the quality of the filling is usually crap).
✗ Sausage rolls, pork-pies, quiche, etc.
✗ Chip-butties, hot-pork sandwich with all the trimmings

Of course, there are hundreds for options for a healthy lunch and who's to say you can't have a bowl of cereal or poached eggs on toast.

Super lunch Plan

LUNCH	Protein	Carbs	Fat	Cals
Salad box: Tomatoes, peppers, cucumber, leaves, onions, etc.	2g	8g	1g	49
Handful of pasta or new potatoes	2g	20g	1g	97
Sandwich: 2 x med slices or 1 x roll on wholemeal bread and lightly buttered (see below for fillings)	8g	38g	15g	319
Deli wrap 10"	5g	30g	5g	185
Med Jacket Potato (dry)	6g	56g	0.5g	245
4 x crisp bread: lightly buttered	4g	24g	10g	210
Fillings for above Cottage cheese: 100g Tuna & mayo:100g Baked beans: 100g Ham (2 x med deli slices) Chicken breast: 100g	13g 20g 7g 16g 25g	3g 4g 20g 4g 0g	4g 15g 1g 9g 1g	100 231 321 117 161
Soup: Scotch broth, veg, etc. 260g tin	4g	24g	1g	121
Soup: cream of tomato, etc. 260g tin	4g	24g	14g	238

Okay, let's see what we can have for dinner (or tea, if you're a Northern person).

*****

Chapter 12:
Evening meal

'There's nothing wrong with 'ready-made' meals, so long as you've put all
the ingredients together and got them ready yourself!
Paul & Ann

THERE ARE far too many options for your evening meal to list here, but the general rule is to - where possible - cut back on a high carb dinner.

Due to something called 'insulin sensitivity', carbs eaten at the end of the day are more likely to be converted into fat than carbs eaten for breakfast or lunch. When you first rise, your muscles and liver cells (the main storage sites for carbs) are more 'sensitive' to insulin. This means they are more likely to accept any recently ingested carbs from the bloodstream. As the day progresses, your fat cells become more 'sensitive' instead; so, potentially, carbs eaten later may convert to fat more easily.

Note: we're saying this is a likelihood, not a definite because the daily energy balance (calories in/out) is paramount. If you've not eaten much in the day and your carb stores are low, then they will still be sensitive and eating carbs in the evening will cause fewer overspills into your fat stores. Exercise depletes carb stores as well and if you've come home from the gym or exercise class the same rule applies.

Most people have regular habits with their evening meals: fish on Monday, chilli-con-carne on Tuesday, chicken on Weds, etc. So, look at making the best options for the foods that you eat week in, week out.

Again, unless you are trying to speed up the weight loss (Chapter 15), don't get overly concerned about something that you eat infrequently, e.g., on birthdays or date-night, etc.

Tip: If you really want a high carb evening meal or have no options due to situations such as eating out or family meals, then either get to the gym or stick to mainly protein foods during the day.

Okay, let's see what's on the evening meal menu

Super

✓ Chicken/turkey breast. All types of fish and shellfish

✓ Any type of meat substitute

✓ All vegetables (frozen is fine)

✓ All pulses and legumes (beans, chick peas, etc.)

Safe

✓ Pork chops, sirloin/rump steak

✓ Lean minced steak. Chicken or Fish in breadcrumbs

✓ New potatoes, rice, couscous and pasta (only one portion: 1 x cupped hand).

✓ Jacket potato (small to medium, without butter)

✓ Sweet potato fries/wedges, etc.

✓ Soups: minestrone, scotch broth, vegetable, etc.

Sneaky

✓ Lamb chops

✓ Burgers (any)

✓ Fish in batter

✓ Chips, onion rings

✓ 'Cream of' soups

✓ Creamy or cheese-based sauces added to pasta, rice, etc.

Scandalous

- ✗ High carb/fat microwave meals: lasagne, etc.
- ✗ Pizza, kebabs and takeaways, especially curries

Super evening meal

(All values are approximate, please check relevant food labels).

EVENING MEAL	Protein	Carbs	Fat	Cals
Salmon fillet & lemon sauce. Small serving new potatoes	22g	12g	12g	244
plus generous portion of broccoli & mange tout	5gg	18g	1g	101
Stir fry chicken breast	25g	2g	2g	126
1 x cup stir fry veg plus 1x cup bean sprouts & soy sauce	4g	10g	4g	236
Quinoa ½ cup (80g)	11g	50g	5g	289
Mediterranean veg	2g	14g	5g	109
Spanish omelette: 2 x eggs	1g	17g	22g	330
Steak sirloin or fillet	40g	0g	7g	223
Small serving oven fries	3g	26g	4g	152
Salad veg	2g	10g	5g	93
Quorn cottage pie	8g	27g	4g	176
2 x serving of veg (broccoli, green beans, peas, carrots, etc)	8g	25g	4g	168

Now, let's see what's great to eat as a snack.

*****

Chapter 13:
Snacks

'You're not a dog, so don't reward yourself for good behaviour with treats.'
Paul & Ann

THE MAIN CRITERION for a good snack is a food that is nutritious, reasonably filling and doesn't give you a sugar spike. There are hundreds of simple snack ideas from wrapping lettuce leaves around tuna, mayo and tomatoes to guacamole on tortilla chips. However, we're going to look at a few that you can simply put in your shopping trolley, keep in the car or buy if you're in a rush.

We think some of the best snack options are:

Fruit

Any type of fruit: apples, bananas, pears, oranges, etc. are good choices but be careful of grapes as they are full of sugar and it's easy to eat loads in one go. Weight for weight, dried fruit is more calorific.

Nuts

Nutrition-wise, almonds, walnuts and Brazil nuts are probably the best option but anything - other than peanuts - are ok. Serving wise, try not to eat more than would just about cover half the palm of your hand. (Yes, we know it's not much, but you can really pile on the calories with nuts.)

Crisp breads/rice cakes

Each maker has its own website with loads of recipe options to choose from with hundreds of toppings, so check a few out and enjoy.

Natural Yoghurts

The following is a list of ingredients taken from a leading brand of a fruit flavoured 'low-fat' yoghurt:

Yoghurt, Water, Black Cherries, (6%), Fructose, Modified Maize Starch, Cocoa Butter, Cocoa Powder, Fat Reduced Cocoa Powder, Butter, Sugar, Stabilisers: Pectins, Guar Gum; Gelatine, Flavourings, Acidity Regulators: Citric Acid, Calcium Citrates; Sodium Citrates, Sweeteners: Aspartame, Acesulfame K, Dark Chocolate Sprinkles (0.4%).

Now the ingredients in natural yoghurt:

Milk, natural live cultures: Bifid bacterium and lactobacillus acidophilus (healthy gut bacteria).

Need we say any more about why you should eat natural yoghurt?

Tip: Stir in a small serving of protein powder, a handful of fresh or frozen berries or some granola to improve taste

Super

✓ All fruit (except grapes)
✓ Crispbreads and rice cakes (or equivalent)
✓ All nuts (except peanuts)
✓ Carrots/celery sticks
✓ Natural, full-fat Greek yoghurt
✓ High protein yoghurts: Quark, Arla, etc.

Safe

✓ Naturally flavoured yoghurt (strawberry, etc.)
✓ Protein shakes

✓ Hummus dip
✓ Mixed nuts & seeds

Sneaky

✓ Yoghurts where you mix in the fruit flavouring
✓ Cereal/protein bars
✓ Trail mix (nuts and dried fruit), peanuts and dry roasted nuts
✓ Ready-made meal replacement drinks

Scandalous

✗ Cakes, biscuits, buns, chocolate bars,
✗ Mini scotch-eggs, pork pies, sausage roll, etc.

Super snacks

(All values are approximate, please check relevant food labels.)

SNACKS	Protein	Carbs	Fat	Cals
Fruit: see breakfast				
Crisp breads: each	1g	6g	0.5g	33
Rice cakes: each	1	5	trace	24
Hummus dip: 2 x tbsp	3g	6g	4g	72
Nuts: various (handful)	5g	4g	12g	144
Greek yoghurt 125g	6g	6g	11g	147
Protein shake in water	22g	4g	3g	211

*****

Chapter 14:
Desserts, oils, spreads & drinks

'Yes, chocolate is made from cocoa, so technically it's a plant.
But no, it's not one of your five a day'
Paul & Ann

OKAY, AFTER READING all this healthy stuff, you're probably desperate to find something yummy. Some delicious-tasting food that explodes on the taste buds but doesn't settle on the hips. Well, let's see if we can rustle-up something for you. If you like to prepare your own food there are some great ideas such as making ice-cream from avocados or dipping a banana in melted dark chocolate, rolling it in coconut flakes and leaving it in the freezer. So, if this is you, simply Google 'low calorie desserts', sit back and enjoy. However, we're going to show you what you can buy from the supermarket.

Desserts

The first thing to understand about desserts is that the calories really pile up when you mix fat and sugar together. So, ideally, keep away from the full-fat cream products and stay with things like crème fraiche, sorbets, light mousses, etc. – and even dark chocolate is not too bad.

Most supermarkets will offer a 'healthy range' of low-fat desserts that use a variety of alternatives to fat. However, this may not reduce the calories because you may find that the sugar content has gone up (remember: sugar can be chemically altered to hold more water, providing a texture, or mouth-feel, to resemble fat), so check the label.

Our advice is that if you eat dessert on a regular basis, make sure you are picking a good option. But if you only eat it on special occasions, don't worry unduly about it.

We can't really offer our usual categories for desserts because there really aren't many that you can class as 'super', and millions that would be sneaky or scandalous. So, we'll just offer a few safer options

Safe (relatively)

✓ Lemon/strawberry mousse
✓ Sorbet
✓ Berries & crème fraiche
✓ Fat-free frozen yoghurt
✓ Fruit salad in juice
✓ Low-fat rice pudding
✓ Low-fat ice cream
✓ Dark chocolate (at least 80% cocoa)

Deserts

DESSERT	Protein	Carbs	Fat	Cals
Mouse: various 125g	2g	12g	6g	110
Sorbet: 125mg	0g	31g	0g	124
Berries and crème fraiche	1g	10g	10g	134
Frozen Yoghurt: 125mg	2g	21g	3g	119
Fruit salad in juice: 125g	1g	16g	0g	40
Low-fat rice pudding 125g	5g	30g	4g	176
Low-fat Ice cream 2 x scoops	4g	16g	6g	134
Dark chocolate: 5 pieces	2g	24g	10g	194

Oils, spreads & condiments

In most cases, it's unlikely that you'll get too many calories from a blob of tomato sauce or a tablespoon of chutney. So, we don't worry about anything extra that is added to improve the taste of your food unless it contains fat or cream. Even then, if it's only a teaspoon of tartar sauce or horseradish, it will hardly break the bank. And the health benefits of oils such as olive or flaxseed far outweigh the calories they supply.

The issue is often not whether the oil has any health benefits but how the one you are buying has been manufactured. For example, many vegetable oils (canola, sunflower, safflower, etc.) are often heated, then treated with petroleum solvents, heated again and flavoured. Doesn't sound too healthy does it?

So, our lists below are assuming that the oil in question has been manufactured responsibly using, where possible, a 'cold-pressed' process. However, if it's for cooking, then heat-pressed will be better because it's less likely to 'burn' at higher cooking temperatures.

The stuff to worry about are things like creamy curry and pasta sauces, applying mayo with a trowel or slathering so much butter on your toast that your arteries are waving the white flag from the first bite. Again, using a small amount of oil to cook with won't be an issue but if you're trying to deep fry your bacon in chip-fat, then you'll have a definite problem. So, before you start to lose sleep over what oil or spread to use, just think about how much you use. If you're buying it every week, then pick the best options; if it's once every other month, don't worry.

Note: current research supports coconut oil as a super food. Chemically, coconut oil is high in saturated fat but it's not the same saturates that are linked with health issues such as diabetes and high cholesterol. It's even thought that this type of saturated fat (called a medium chain triglyceride or MCT) will improve health and it may be the latest 'super-must-have-food' to hit the market.

But, we're going to keep an eye on this and see how it develops. Incidentally, coconut water is rubbish. It's about as close to a proper coconut as we are to the West Indies (we're in Sheffield).

To be honest, we've spent hours trying to research the topic of healthy oils and it's almost impossible to find a list that everyone agrees with. However, let's offer our advice (but we're sure someone will disagree) and we're assuming you will use these products as sparingly as possible.

Super

- ✓ Oils: olive, flaxseed, avocado, sesame, walnut,
- ✓ Coconut oil/butter
- ✓ Fish oils: omega 3, 6 & 9
- ✓ Proper butter (from grass-fed cows)

Safe

- ✓ Sunflower oil
- ✓ Basmati
- ✓ Soy sauce
- ✓ Tomato or brown sauce
- ✓ Chutneys and pickles
- ✓ Olive or sunflower oil-based butter alternatives

Sneaky

- ✓ Palm oil, canola oil
- ✓ Ghee
- ✓ Safflower oil
- ✓ Margarine
- ✓ Creamy sauces for pasta, curry, etc.

Scandalous

- ✗ Cheap cooking oil
- ✗ Anything that contains the word 'hydrogenated'

Drinks

Where do we start with drinks? It's unlikely that fat will account for the calories (except for milk-based smoothies). So, the culprit will be sugar and boy, can it be a problem. Don't think that just because it's in liquid form it's automatically low-calorie. We had a client that drink tea all day long and each cup had milk and two sugars. This accounted for almost 1,000k/cals per day! So, if you're not careful, you can pile on the calories with sugary drinks and without exception, they are all empty calories.

We've put together a quick list to offer a few options and we'll look at alcohol in chapter 16.

Super

✓ Water

✓ Tea: green, camomile, herbal & fruit teas

✓ Coffee (black). Coffee doesn't suit everyone but there's plenty of evidence that it can have some very beneficial properties in limited doses

Safe

✓ All other types of tea with milk (no sugar)

✓ Coffee with milk (instant, filter, americano, espresso, etc.)

✓ Diluted cordials (no added sugar)

Sneaky

✓ All forms of fresh or carton fruit juice

✓ Isotonic sports drinks

✓ Caffeinated energy drinks – even the sugar free versions

Scandalous

✗ Popular-branded fizzy drinks, including diet versions (see artificial sweeteners in chapter 16)

- ✗ Coffee: large servings from popular chain outlets that have been sweetened with syrups and contain full-fat milk. Some of these drinks can contain over 700k/cals.
- ✗ Volcanic bottled water (or similar from undisturbed fjords in Sweden, etc.). These are only scandalous because they are a complete rip-off and offer absolutely no health benefits other than making your wallet a lot lighter.
- ✗ Incidentally, most bottled water is only tap water that's been run through a filter by the maker.

Okay, let's see if we can speed up the weight loss a little.

*****

Chapter 15:
Faster results

'Burn 1,200 calories in a minute – set fire to your pizza!'
Paul & Ann

HOPEFULLY, YOU have now realised that the best way to win the inch war is a nice, steady weight loss regime that includes healthy eating. But what if you want to get faster results? How do you lose weight a bit quicker without upsetting your metabolism, making yourself ill or suffering from a serious weight-gain-rebound? (Remember Chapter 2: As fat as a pig!) Obviously, one way is to increase and maintain high levels of activity (we'll cover the best way to do this in book 2), but what about your diet?

Let's look at some options.

Clean up your diet

The first thing to consider is that it's not necessarily a matter of how much you need to do, but how little can you get away with and still succeed. Basically, this means don't do everything at once. Don't start running marathons and living off nettle soup from day one. It's amazing just how much weight you can lose by little more than cutting out the junk.

So, your first task is simple: clean up your diet and increase your daily activity.

For example:

- ✓ Cut back on the treats, pastries, crisps, alcohol. Make them a treat, not a staple food. If you must have them, then earn them with extra activity.
- ✓ Eat wraps instead of sandwiches, mini rice cakes instead of crisps, plain biscuits instead of chocolate ones, spritzers instead of wine, etc.
- ✓ If you're having a high fat meal, don't have a lot of starchy carbs.
- ✓ If you're going out for a meal in the evening, stick to '**super**' foods or protein only during the day, likewise if you've had a big night out, do the same the following day.

All these things help, and they are just great habits to get into because it's tricks like these that not only help you to lose weight but stop it piling back on.

Now, we're going to show you how we help our clients to speed up the weight loss without impacting their metabolic rate.

Feast and famine?

Varying your calorie intake from one day to another is a highly effective method of losing weight. It's not a new idea; in fact, it's been around for ages. It's also known as feast and famine (but you'll need avoid the feast part if you want to speed up the weight loss). And it was popularised recently as the 5:2 Diet, or Intermittent Fasting (IF).

If you've not already heard of the 5:2 Diet, it's a very simple idea. For two days per week, you only eat about 400-500 calories per day, preferably all in your evening meal. For the other five days, it's alleged you can 'eat what you want'.

Sorry, but this another claim that is utter nonsense. There are definite health benefits to not eating much for a few days, the primary one being improved insulin sensitivity (which is vital if you're carrying a considerable amount of abdominal fat).

But calorie-wise, if you starve yourself of food one day and stuff your face to busting point the next, you will, at best, not lose any weight and at worst, get fatter - energy in versus energy out is the primary law of weight loss/gain.

Despite not being overly enthusiastic about any diet that promotes starving over eating better, we like this idea and it works very well in short bursts. But bear in mind this is not really a diet, as it's simply not eating for two days out of every seven. However, one of the best things it does is to teach you that being hungry is not life-threatening.

Tip: Hunger pangs come in waves that last for about 10-15 minutes and once you accept them - that you're only hungry - and not actually starving to death, you finally learn to have greater control of your eating habits.

The downside with it is that it can become tedious after a while and increasingly difficult to fit into your life, as it's an all or nothing plan. For example, you pick two, non-consecutive days to fast and Monday is usually the first one (after the weekend's excess). You then decide which day will be the best for the next fast, but life often interferes with your plans. Thursday may be the best option but you're meeting friends for a drink after work that day. Tuesday is out as it's too close to Monday, so maybe Wednesday is best. Nope, no good, you've got a business lunch scheduled.

What about Friday? Friday looks ideal, until Thursday comes along, and you suddenly get an invite to a birthday party or your boss sends you out of town on business for the day and you realise you can't possible drive 300 miles up and down the motorway on an empty stomach.

Unless you have the social calendar of a leper, trying to fast at the weekend is futile, so it's start all over again on Monday. All or nothing eating plans don't last because they are not consistent - you're either fully on the diet or you're not - and to effectively shift your body fat, and keep it off, you must be consistent.

We have a couple of other options which we think work better.

1. The 16-hour fast

This is another version of intermittent fasting that only allows you to eat within an eight-hour window. From your last meal in the evening, you can't eat for the next 16-hours. Obviously, you'll need to drink, so water is fine, and we also drink tea or coffee (milk is okay but no sugar). Therefore, if your last meal was 7pm, you can't eat any more food until 1pm the following day. Also, if you keep to 'super' and 'safe' foods during the remaining eight-hour window, you'll stay full and keep your calories low.

The safe maximum number of fasting days you can have per week is five, spread out over the week as your lifestyle dictates. Start with just two or three 16-hour fasting days and increase or decrease as necessary.

Tip: If you don't think you could cope without eating first thing, then try a carbs-free breakfast. For example, just have a couple of boiled eggs, because this will keep your insulin levels low and not defeat the object of the fast.

2. Calorie cycling

This involves varying the calorie intake from day to day, again as your lifestyle dictates. The brilliance of this regime is it stops your body from adapting to a specific energy intake and if you don't go too low, too often, you will avoid the weight loss plateau.

Option A: count calories

For those of you who want to use calories as your gauge, you need to calculate how many calories you burn off daily. If you want a rough idea, first convert your weight into pounds (1kg=2.2lbs). Then, multiply this figure by twelve for men, or ten for women. This provides a rough calculation for an 'average' man or woman with a fairly sedentary lifestyle. **Don't add on the calories burnt from activity or exercise because you want to use these extra calories to add towards your deficit.**

Once you have this number - for argument's sake, let's say it's 2,000 calories – you then convert this into a total weekly amount: 7 x 2,000 = 14,000k/cals.

Now, we need to make some sort of deficit in this figure. We usually aim to start with about a 20% cut (2,800 calories), which reduces the weekly calorie allowance to approximately 11,000 calories. You can always cut back a bit more later but remember, don't do too much too soon. If necessary, increase your activity to burn off a bit more. Your objective is not to eat more than 11,000 calories throughout the week.

Rather than simply dividing this figure by seven, you could try three days at 2,000; two days at 1,500 and two days at 1,000 calories. The permutations are entirely up to you.

Tip: You can use this system in conjunction with the 16-hour fast to help reduce your weekly calorie balance. However, don't overdo the low-calorie days because you'll defeat the object of the diet.

Option B: control your carbs

The other option is to ignore calories and use our Super, Safe and Sneaky food options. Again, using permutations to suit you, vary between days where you only eat 'super' foods; days when you have 'super' and 'safe' foods, and days where you add in some 'sneaky' foods. This is basically controlling your carb intake because all super and safe foods are high in protein and low in starchy carbs.

For a long-term plan, this is our recommended option because fasting sometimes has the tendency to create sugar cravings as a reward for not eating. You know the ones: those, 'I've been really good all day, so I can afford to be really bad tonight' urges that arrive at the end of a stressful day.

To be honest, there are no perfect options and we can pick spots off every plan, including our own. Our experience tells us that plans such as IF and calorie cycling work well for most people because they are flexible, not only regarding what you can eat but also when you can eat it.

This allows you to fit the diet into your life and not the other way around. Therefore, it offers your new eating plan a greater chance of success.

Important warnings:

1. We do not recommend that you extend any form of continuous calorie cycling beyond 30 days. Attempting to lose weight rapidly by fasting is not a safe practice. To avoid both damage to your metabolism and health, apply equal amounts of time dieting with normal eating. For example, diet for one month, then eat normally (as per the general recommendations in this book) for the next. Then repeat if necessary.
2. Do not undertake this type of plan if you are pregnant or breast-feeding. Nor if you are prone to, or have a history of, eating disorders (bulimia, binge-eating, etc.), mood swings, depression, etc. Fasting can interfere with some medications, so please contact your GP or local health practitioner first.

Okay, we've talked at length about the types of food to eat but what about the rest of the important stuff that may be useful to know when you start your weight loss regime?

So, it's time to see what's leftover.

*****

Chapter 16:

Leftovers

'Boiling water softens potatoes but hardens eggs. So, it's not the situation but what you do with it that counts'.
Paul & Ann

OKAY, YOU'VE endured a Domestic Science lesson on nutrition, read about macros and micros, sorted a food diary out, looked over the super eating plans and hopefully now have good plan formulating in your head. However, we've not quite finished with you yet. In this part of the book, we're going to very cover some of the topics that fall into the 'some useful stuff you really need to know'. There's a lot to cover, so we've just added a quick list below so that you can read it all or just pick a topic that may be of interest.

Alcohol

Alcohol is not a food calorie, it's a toxin (poison). However, your body can use both the alcohol and sugar content of your favourite tipple as energy. Unfortunately, this is where calculating its energy value gets a bit tricky. First, some of the alcohol you consume is lost via breath, sweat and urine. Then, it loses between 20-30% of its energy value[4] as it's processed by the liver (possibly more if you're drinking on an empty stomach). Finally, because everyone processes alcohol differently, it's very difficult to determine the net calorie value from one person to another. But this doesn't mean that you can go out and get smashed whenever you want because it has some very negative effects. It will:

- ✓ Reduce sleep quality
- ✓ Increase insulin resistance
- ✓ Promote fat storage around the belly
- ✓ Elevate oestrogen levels in men (and makes them think they can fight like Conan the Barbarian and dance like John Travolta – often both in the same evening)
- ✓ Increase appetite
- ✓ Suppresses your natural fat burning capacity

If you want to lose weight, then alcohol is definitely not your friend. If you can't give up a glass of wine or a bottle of beer for just two or three days of the week or cannot seem to have any control over the amount you drink, then your alcohol intake will impact on your weight loss targets. **Our policy is that there's often no need to stop drinking, just stop drinking as much**.

Tip: To save calories, try vodka and slimline tonic or a white wine spritzer (with a low-sugar lemonade or soda).

Artificial sweeteners

Artificial sweeteners are also known as sugar substitutes. They are low-calorie or calorie-free chemical substances that are used instead of sugar to sweeten foods and drinks. Despite rigorous testing and claims of no side-effects by such agencies as UK Cancer Research and the European Food Safety Authority, we are wary of these products.

Most artificial sweeteners are used by the diet drink or diet soda industry and this is where we have serious concerns. Drinks manufacturers claim there are no side-effects from their products but type 'diet drink addiction' in Google and you get nearly 30 million hits!

Some of the stories are frightening, with many people consuming up to eight litres of 'diet drinks' per day! Much of the problem could be down to the high amounts of caffeine they generally contain, but it's more likely the effect they have on your brain.

Evolution has hard-wired our brains to love sugar for its instant-energy hit, which was often vital for survival. In nature, sugar is only found in any reasonable quantities in fruit. But the sweeter the fruit, the higher the sugar content, hence our ingrained love for sweet, fruity-tasting food and drink.

The problem

The instant sugar hits your tongue, signals fly to the brain telling it that sugar is coming. Then, your pancreas pumps insulin into the bloodstream to lower your blood sugar levels in expectation of the incoming energy (which could potentially raise blood sugar to dangerous levels). However, herein lays the problem: with diet drinks, there is no energy - it's like receiving a blank cheque when you were expecting your wages.

The brain kicks-off: "Where's my sugar"' it demands, as the recent hormonal shift has lowered blood sugar levels and they are now falling rapidly enough to make you feel light-headed.

So, you either reach out for other quick-sugar-fix foods such as chocolate or biscuits, or even worse, you have another diet drink and the cycle continues. This is the reason why diet drinks can be addictive: they promise much but provide nothing in the way of satisfaction. And it's the constant seeking of satisfaction that creates the addiction[*].

The answer

Wean yourself off them. Replace them with plain water. If you really want a bit of taste, add a squeeze of natural lemon juice. If you drink multiple cans per day, start with one replacing one can per day for a week, then two, then three, etc., until you've ditched them completely.

Detox supplements/products

Let's get one thing unarguably, indefatigably clear: there is absolutely no scientific evidence[5] behind any of these products and study after study has shown they are simply not necessary.

Your liver and kidneys are perfectly designed to detoxify your body, if you just give them the chance. Just stop taking the toxic products - alcohol, caffeine, processed foods, etc. - then eat plenty of fruit and natural veg and drink lots of water for about 5-7days and you've got an instant detox system.

We can't however, deny the 'placebo' effect of such products. In some cases, people need to 'draw a line in the sand' e.g. that was my old lifestyle, and this is my new one, using a 'detox' plan to bridge the gap between the two.

We wouldn't argue too hard against this thinking because as we keep saying, you've got to find something that works for you.

------

[*] *It can get worse. Some of these sweeteners also act as mild laxatives, so not only can you become dizzy, you also get the runs, which is a nightmare-scenario that will never end well*

Just make sure that if you do 'detox', you're doing it for the right reasons, otherwise, you will simply be throwing your money away.

Free radicals & anti-oxidants

A free radical is microscopic, toxic compound that's produced whenever oxygen is used by our cells, which is pretty much all of them – all the time! They are basically scavengers that will try to disrupt healthy cells and they are neutralised by other compounds called anti-oxidants. If they are not neutralised, they cause the early death of healthy cells and are closely linked to increases in all forms of cancers and heart disease.

You may not be aware of it, but your body is producing thousands of damaging free radicals every second. If you smoke, drink a lot of alcohol, live in a built-up area, eat highly processed foods, then you will increase your production of free radicals through the inhalation of pollutants and ingestion of more toxic compounds.

Other than living like a monk on a desert island, the best way to combat free radicals is to increase your intake of foods that not only contain high levels of anti-oxidants but also promote the production of our body's natural anti-oxidants.

These are the ones that we think are the best.

Salmon & Mackerel

✓ Fresh is better than tinned and is a fantastic source of healthy fish oils. Try not to eat the skin of any fish as it has likely to have absorbed any pollutants in the water where the fish are caught. Salmon is often farmed, and this has led to some health scares and questions as to the quality of the fish due to the 'fish food' it is fed, so make sure it's wild Pacific or Atlantic

Avocados

✓ Full of natural anti-oxidants and omega oils

Cottage cheese

✓ Excellent source of Tryptophan, an amino acid vital to produce the hormone serotonin (your 'happy' hormone)

Broccoli, water cress, kale & spinach

✓ Fantastic source of vitamins and minerals, especially iron

Nuts: Almonds, Brazil nuts, walnuts and cashew (not peanuts).

✓ Good source of proteins, iron, healthy fats and fibre

Seeds: Flax, pumpkin, sunflower, etc.

✓ Good source of proteins, healthy fats, zinc, iron and fibre

Tomatoes

✓ Natural cancer fighting anti-oxidants

Linseed/Flaxseed Oil

✓ Great source of natural omega 3 oils

Fruit

✓ All fruits are brilliant but the best, from an anti-oxidant and health point would be the citrus fruits: oranges, lemons, etc. - and the daddy of them all is the Kiwi fruit

Irritable bowel syndrome

Irritable bowel syndrome (IBS) is becoming more common in today's world. Firstly, diagnosing and treating IBS is beyond the scope of this book and something that we will leave to the medical profession. However, not everything that presents as a common symptom of IBS: bloating, cramps, gas, etc., is, in fact, a medical problem. Often, it's dietary induced and this is a little bit easier to deal with if you know what to look for. (Incidentally, a recent study[6] showed that 86% of people who think they are intolerant to gluten, actually are not). Whilst you think you have gluten intolerance, you may in fact, suffer from SIBO or FODMAPS.

SIBO & FODMAPS

SIBO[7] stands for Small Intestinal Bacterial Overgrowth and FODMAPS[8] is Fermentable Oligosaccharides, Disaccharides, Monosaccharides and Polyols. Both are conditions that will present as IBS, but the causes can be quite different and possibly simpler to treat. Basically, you must look at your sugar intake (another reason for doing a food diary).

There are approximately one hundred trillion (100,000,000,000) bacteria in your gut that are vital for digestion. We have a symbiotic relationship with these bacteria: our food feeds them and they, in turn, break food down and help to process vital nutrients for us to absorb. If you didn't have them, you would die of malnutrition.

However, not all the bacteria are the same and some perform different duties to others and the ones that cause SIBO/FODMAPS happen to love sugar. In a healthy gut they usually don't get chance to feast on it because they live in the lower intestine (colon) and sugar gets absorbed in the upper intestine.

Their job is to help process soluble and non-soluble fibre before it leaves the body and a side effect of this work is gas - a build-up of which is often expelled prior to the bowel being evacuated.

If you have SIBO/FODMAPS, these bacteria have managed to migrate up the intestine and are now feasting on sugar. This means the gas has a long, long way to go to get out and as the small intestine is tightly packed behind the stomach, the pressure causes not only discomfort but extreme abdominal distension (swollen belly) as well - in some cases making you look six months pregnant!

SIBO/FODMAPS is often caused by (but not exclusively) prolonged alcohol and caffeine consumption and the most common symptom (apart from bloating) is excessive flatulence. It is treatable by antibiotics but cutting back on all sugars - especially the simple sugars from fruit, biscuits, etc. - for two weeks may be the first thing to try. Your GP should be able to perform a simple test if this hasn't had any effect[*].

Testing for intolerances

Whilst we are discussing intolerances, etc., it's worth noting there are several companies in the UK offering all sorts of food intolerance tests. Our advice would be to ignore them. The only person you should consult is your doctor, who can arrange proper, medical tests. In our experience, everyone we've talked to who've had over the counter tests have invariably been told they are intolerant to wheat, dairy and red food colouring (and peas for some strange reason).

We've lost count of how many times we've heard some celebrity Personal Trainer claim that their client has lost weight purely because of the 'cleansing detox' by cutting out alcohol, coffee, meat, wheat & dairy (and peas) from their diet. That's not a diet, it's just not eating anything!

---

[*] *On the plus side, the excess flatulence from SIBO & FOMAPS may increase calorie expenditure, as you'll always have to take the stairs, instead of the lift! Always think positive.*

In most cases just cutting wheat & dairy alone from your diet will account for about an overnight 40-50% drop in calories, so it's not surprising that you lose weight. Whilst cutting back or cutting out alcohol and caffeine is never a bad idea (as they have no real nutritional value) wheat and dairy do, such as calcium from milk or the Vitamin B range from wheat bran and zinc from yeast, etc. If you cut these foods out, then you're going to have to ensure you replace the lost vitamins and minerals with something else (and just reaching for a bottle of multi-vits is a cop-out).

Remember, food intolerances are often dose related, so you may not have to cut them out, just cut them back. Initially, a simple way to check any problems is to cut out one food at a time that you think is causing the problem for at least seven days and see what happens. If the symptoms reduce or stop altogether, then you know you're on the right lines.

Now, this is important, reintroduce it slowly back into your diet and see if the symptoms reoccur. If they do, you can be pretty sure you've got the right food and now it's a case of finding out how much you can tolerate before the symptoms become intolerable[*].

Allergies and intolerances are tricky subjects for laypeople like us to discuss and we've only included this section to highlight potential problems with food. Don't take our word as gospel and if you have concerns and if you don't want to see your doctor/GP first, check out the Food Standards Agency, NHS or other such Government organisation for further information.

---

[*] *Strangely enough, we find we can cope with about three glasses of wine before we suddenly become very intolerant to it – weird, huh!*

Reformed food

Following on from the food chain there is a type of meat which is so far down the chain, it's almost a missing link!

No one likes wasting food, especially food manufacturers and if there's money to be made from scraps, they'll bend over backwards to get it. Reformed food or Mechanically Reclaimed Meat (MRM) covers a range of methods (multitude of sins?) to get every particle of food from a cow, pig, lamb, chicken or fish.

So, let's have a quick look at the various ways they reclaim the scraps

Meat glue

Food manufacturers use a perfectly legal chemical called transglutaminase (you can even buy it from Amazon) to stick scraps of meat together. And because it's classed as a 'processing aid' not an ingredient, it doesn't need to be on the label. Basically, offcuts of meat are thrown into a vat. The transglutaminase is added, it's given a good stir and left for a few hours. Enzymes in the transglutaminase act as glue that bind the proteins together until finally, you have a solid lump of meat and fat. This is then formed into a variety of shapes to resemble traditional cuts of meat. Now, we can't claim there's a health issue with this process, but it's a bit sneaky. And unfortunately, it doesn't always end here because the product can also be 'padded out' with other, dubious bits of an animal.

Acid bath

All the inedible and unused bits of the animal – skin, bones, intestines, etc. – are placed in large vat. Phosphates (acids) are also added to dissolve the protein in meat, removing it from the bones, gristle, skin, etc. Everything is then spun in a centrifuge to separate the meat from the rest. The residue, known as meat slurry, is naturally sticky, allowing it to bind to water, which also increases its weight. Again, flavours and colourings are added so that it resembles meat.

Soya

Soya flour or 'protein isolate' is often added to stretch the meat content out further. Incidentally, adding this isolate to any food is a popular way of increasing its protein content.

Gelatine

Gelatine is the skin, cartilage, ligaments and other connective tissues of an animal. Watching the process of creating gelatine (also known as hydrolysed collagen) is almost guaranteed to turn the most avid meat lover into a staunch vegetarian. This can also be coloured to resemble meat and again, often added to the mix. So yes, the label may say 80% beef or pork, but actually how much of it is originally from the edible parts of the animal is questionable.

Formed from and reformed

In general, meat that is 'Formed from' is usually more expensive and indicates that better cuts have been used. However, 'reformed from' could be anything. Reformed meat often ends up as 'wafer thin' slices of ham or beef and it's very common in cheap sausages, burger and mince.

Tip: Food manufacturers must state all the ingredients of the product on its food label. The list starts with the main constituents (by volume) first and descends to the least. If hydrolysed collagen, gelatine, trimmings, etc. are anywhere near the top of the list, don't buy it (unless of course, you fancy eating an animal's mucky bits). If you shop in a supermarket, try to buy your meat from a deli-counter because they must state whether the meats are formed or natural cuts and if you're not sure, you can ask.

Weight-loss supplements

The supplement industry is very clever at creating a problem that doesn't exist and then selling you a solution that you didn't need in the first place. And the makers of weight-loss aids are masters of their nefarious art.

Most weight loss supplements come in three basic types: fat burner, appetite suppressant or fat blocker. In later chapters, we'll examine the myths surrounding your body's limited capacity to burn fat, but for now, we'll try to keep it simple and make just a few comments.

- ✓ If they are so good, why do they all state: **only effective as part of a calorie-controlled diet?** And why aren't they offered by the NHS? Surely, a course of tablets is more cost effective than a gastric band?
- ✓ The more effective the product, then the greater the side effects. This includes headaches, palpitations, insomnia, panic attacks and diarrhoea amongst many, many others. Not to mention that many are also highly addictive. Often, once you start down the diet-pill path, it's hard to turn back.
- ✓ Taking a fat loss supplement that blocks fat absorption is like taking an aspirin for the headache you've just got from banging your head against a brick wall. If you don't bang your head in the first place, you won't need the pain-killer. Take control of your life and stop eating the stuff that's making you fat and you won't need the tablets.
- ✓ Having the fat microwaved or lasered off still entails undertaking a 40-minute treadmill session to burn the fat off afterwards. And the claims by the Raspberry Ketone brigade that you can 'cleave' fat cells must rate as the biggest load of nonsense we've ever heard.
- ✓ Incidentally, 'diet' foods are only lower calorie versions of normal food with a couple of ingredients, such as green tea or conjugated lineic acid (CLA), thrown in to make them sound special.
- ✓ Regardless of whatever the supplement may claim, the effects can only be minimal; you've still got to get your diet right and do some exercise.

The health halo

Incidentally, it's worth pointing out that just because you've decided to eat more healthily, it doesn't mean you will still lose weight. Recent studies are laying some of the blame for the western world's rising obesity levels down to something called the Health Halo Effect[9]. It's been well proven that in restaurants, diners picking the 'healthy' options, not only eat bigger portions but order more sides and extras as well.

We've said this once and we'll keep on saying it: the energy balance equation is the primary factor in weight loss (even though is it difficult to calculate). Regardless of the fact that your healthy meal increases the thermic effect of food (TEF) or provides every essential nutrient you need, it still has a calorie value. There is no such thing as a calorie-free meal - healthy or not!

The final few crumbs

To finish with, we just want to cover a few tricks that we use ourselves and have passed on to our clients with great success.

- ✓ If you get a chocolate urge or any type of craving, then go and clean your teeth or rinse with mouth wash (it's the thought of putting chocolate in your mouth after cleaning your teeth – ugh).
- ✓ Another little trick with urges: look at the clock and say to yourself, "If I still want that chocolate bar in 20mins, I'll have it then". Often, by the time 20mins has passed, so has the urge.
- ✓ If you love ice cream, then buy low-fat, frozen yoghurt instead (a client of ours promised to leave us money in his Will when we put him onto this one).

During digestion, your stomach sends out a variety of hormones to tell the brain that food is coming and reports on how full your stomach is.

Unfortunately, it takes the 'I'm now stuffed' signal about 15 minutes to get your brain; subsequently, you can still feel hungry even when the stomach is full.

You can avoid this with the following:

- ✓ Chew your food more slowly and try to use both sides of your mouth to chew with.   Digestion starts in the mouth where food is mechanically broken up and mixed with enzymes in your saliva to help chemically break the food down, making it easier for the stomach to handle. If you don't chew properly, your stomach will take longer to digest your food. This is especially true for carbohydrates, which, if not chewed properly, will start to ferment in the gut, causing intestinal bloating and excess wind

- ✓ Try and put your knife or fork back on the plate whilst chewing and occasionally sip a glass of water between mouthfuls. This means it takes longer to eat your meal and again, improves digestion. Also, the water will contribute to the feeling of satiety (feeling full).

- ✓ Eat a piece of fruit about ten minutes **before** your meal. This starts the digestive processes, reducing the 'I'm now stuffed' signal to the brain, down to about five minutes. If you then eat a little slower, you won't overeat as easily.

- ✓ Incidentally, fruit digests much better on an empty stomach, rather than a full one as the sugar in fruit ferments very easily. Therefore, eating fruit **after** a meal may leave you feeling bloated and full of wind

Okay, that's us just about done for this part about food and diet. Now it's time to consider how your body deals with losing weight. So, we'll have a quick visit to the world of calories, metabolism and stress, then it's straight into understanding the vital role of exercise in a successful, life-long weight loss plan.

*****

Chapter 17:
It's never as simple as it seems

For every complex problem, there is an answer that is simple,
obvious - and wrong!"
H L Mencken

AT FIRST glance, the answer to a successful weight loss plan is obvious: you just eat less and move more. Over the years we've heard this cliché on many, many occasions (generally from people who've never had a weight problem and therefore aren't qualified to comment). Yet, if you suggest this to anyone who struggles with their weight, they'll usually give a humourless little snort, followed by a dour "I wish".

In truth, the eat less/move more solution does work. Without doubt, it's the essential foundation of pretty much every successful weight-loss plan. The problem lies in the context of applying a generalised, overly simple solution to an incredibly complex and individualised problem. Because it's this individuality, i.e. you as a unique person, that's at the heart of the matter.

Where, for example, in the immense scope of eating less and moving more are you? Will not putting sugar in your morning cuppa and taking the stairs instead of the lift at work suffice? Or, do you need to live on nettle soup and run marathons? Believe us, there's a 'sweet spot' for you in there somewhere - it's just a case of finding it.

Ultimately, only you can put these things in context for yourself.

After all, you know yourself better than anyone else and with the right type of map and a set of clear instructions you can decide for yourself how much less is less and how much more is more.

We'll come back to this idea later but for now we need to look at something else that is not what it seems, the cunning calorie.

Tip: We've said this earlier, but it's worth repeating. Always take the path of least resistance to achieve your goals. Don't think, 'how much to I need to do' but consider instead, 'how little can I can get away with and still succeed?' The journey may take a little longer but it's likely to be more enjoyable.

The cunning calorie

The energy (calorie) in/out equation is an elemental function of the universe. It falls under the laws of thermodynamics which arrived with the big bang nearly fourteen billion years ago and will keep going until time itself ends. Magic has no role in its workings, nor does wishful thinking - it's fact. It's the common denominator in every diet in the world. We don't care what diet you talk about, we'll show you how, regardless of any claims to the contrary, it will ultimately reduce your energy intake to less than your expenditure.

On our website there is a spoof newspaper article entitled The Marshmallow Diet, where we prove that eating marshmallows aids weight loss. It was a micky-take on the principle of a two-week diet of replacing normal breakfast and lunch meals with meal-replacement drinks or cereals bars, etc. We demonstrated that because five jumbo-sized marshmallows contain the same calories as the drinks and cereals, the outcome would be exactly the same. We showed that any weight lost is not due to the product itself, but because you've been eating very little food for a fortnight.

However, calorie calculations share the same ambivalent issues as eating less and moving more. Not only are they more complicated than you may think, they are at times, a pointless exercise.

First, however, an explanation of the humble calorie is necessary.

The world has gone calorie mad

Everyone 'rabbits on' about calories. How many in this, how many in that or the other. But what is a calorie - just what are they talking about? It's very confusing: are there fat calories, thin calories, large or small calories? Do calories hate you; do they lie, using cunning and subterfuge to make you fat? Unfortunately, the answer is slightly dull.

In the same way that a ruler measures distance, calories measure energy. **In fact, one Calorie is the amount of energy required to raise the temperature of one litre of water by one degree Celsius**.

Note: One Calorie, with a capital C is equal to one k/cal or one thousand calories (small c).

So, a 'calorie' is just a man-made term to tell you how much energy is being used to make something hotter. So, if you truly think that calories hate you, then you need more help than we can offer. However, if you think they are lying to you, then you're not wrong. Let's see why.

✓ The calorie values found on food labels are not accurate. In the early 1900s, American research chemist Wilbur Atwater first determined the energy-per-gram values of proteins (4k/cals), carbohydrates (4k/cals) and fats (9k/cals). Yet, he admitted that when testing, for example, the same types of apples, he got up to a 20% plus or minus variation. Regardless, the food industry accepted these 'average' figures and now all modern food labelling is a simple matter of multiplying the weight of the ingredients by their relevant 'average' calorie values. So, a 500k/cals meal could be as low as 400k/cals or as much as 600k/cals.

There's more.

✓ Although the food may be in your stomach, it doesn't mean that your body gets to use all of it. In the same way that you have gross pay (before tax, NI, etc.) and net pay (after deductions), you also have gross and net calories. Again, let's see why.

✓ Not all the food you eat will be absorbed into your body. Unprocessed or raw foods are harder to digest than processed foods (processing often does some of the digestive process for you). This can reduce the available amount of both energy and nutrition before it passes out of the system. Also, it takes more energy to digest proteins and vegetables than simple sugars and fats. In the case of protein, your body 'spends' as much as thirty calories of energy to process one hundred calories-worth of protein. Whereas simple sugars and fats only cost about five calories per hundred.

✓ Your metabolism shifts the goalposts when calories drop. **So, there's little point in cutting back on 500k/cals per day if you do it in such a way that your metabolic rate reduces by the same amount**. We'll show you how to avoid this in the next chapter.

✓ Whilst there are some fancy equations involved in the calculation of your energy expenditure, it's often little more than a guess. For example, the equations won't account for high stress levels, poor sleep patterns, recent diet history, menopause, etc. - any of which can reduce your metabolic rate by up to 40%.

Our advice with calories is only use them in terms of comparisons. For example, picking a lower calorie food over a higher one. Or comparing your current calorie intake with what is happening to your body in terms of weight loss or weight gain. We understand this advice likely goes against everything you've ever known but if you rely on calories as your only ally in the weight-loss war, you may as well start measuring your waistline with an elastic tape measure.

Note: our only real exception to counting calories is if we are using a short-term calorie cycling plan.

So, there's no problem with keeping track of your calorie intake, just be aware that calories are not the 'be all and end all' of weight loss.

And don't slavishly follow the amounts set by your friendly phone app, website or any other form of calculation[*].

In the next chapter, we'll show you that permanent weight loss has far more to do with your hormones and metabolic rate than it does with calories, so let's give your metabolism a quick check-up.

*****

---

[*] *It's proven that religiously counting calories increases your chances of developing CDO. (CDO is the advanced stage of OCD – it has the letters in the correct alphabetical order!)*

Chapter 18:
Metabolic mayhem

*'Revving up the metabolic engine is preferable to
just stamping on the calorie brakes'*
Paul & Ann

IF YOU'VE tried to lose weight in the past, you'll know that it rarely follows a straight line. The weight comes off nicely for a couple of weeks, then nothing for a week, then it's dropping again, then either nothing again or it even goes up … before dropping again. This is perfectly natural; it's only the ebb and flow of the hormones that control how your body uses energy (burns fat) and retains or releases water.

However, if you don't keep your metabolism in tip-top running condition, weight loss is either slow, or worse, it grinds permanently to a halt and you hit the dreaded 'plateau'. At which point your odds of winning the inch war are about the same as the Queen abdicating and giving the throne to Posh and Becks! So, let's have a quick look at why this happens and then we'll show you how to avoid the weight-loss merry-go-round.

First, we'll describe how your body adapts to a prolonged, low-calorie diet with a four-phase adaptive process:

1. Acceptance:

For the first two weeks your body accepts the deficit and there's little or no change to your metabolic rate. If you resume normal eating, your metabolism returns to normal immediately.

2. Fight back:

After two weeks of a continuous, low-calorie intake, the fight-back begins. Temporary changes in hormonal balance will force your metabolism to resist the continuing calorie deficit by reducing your usual metabolic rate to preserve your essential fat stores. The rate of weight loss is starting to slow down. If you resume normal eating, your metabolism usually returns to normal within one month.

3. Stalemate:

After about three months of continuous low calories, your metabolic rate is virtually at stalemate with your energy intake. Whilst it assumes the situation may still be temporary, it's adapted to the low-calorie intake. To make up any further calorie shortfall it may prioritise converting muscle tissue to energy rather than body fat. This leads to elevated levels of cortisol and other pro-inflammatory hormones which, in turn, negatively affect the immune system and digestion. If you resume normal eating, your metabolism may return to normal within six to twelve weeks.

4. Surrender:

After about six months of continuous low calories, your metabolism has accepted the reduced calorie intake as normal. Whilst it's still making energy savings and burning off muscle tissue, any temporary hormonal changes have now become permanent and weight loss may have stopped. This phase is commonly referred to as 'famine' mode (the term is rather imprecise, but apt). If you resume normal eating, your metabolism could take between nine to twelve months to recover. But in some cases, it may never fully return to normal.

Note: These are just general timescales and effects and not everyone will suffer them to the same degree, but hopefully, you get the basic idea. Also, the more weight you carry (even if it's fat), the higher your metabolic rate. Therefore, as you get lighter your 'normal' metabolic rate falls respectively.

So, you can see how important it is to keep your metabolic rate in tip-top condition and running nicely, but how do you keep control?

What controls the metabolism?

You have a complex balance of glands* and hormones that regulate your metabolic rate. But ultimately, it's your thyroid gland that's the 'boss' in charge of energy output. It pumps out a couple of hormones (commonly known as T3 and T4) in direct response to your body's current food intake and energy expenditure. To put it simply, your thyroid gland is the metabolic-pointy-stick that prods every cell in your body into action.

Levels of T3 and T4 are high when food is aplenty, and drop following a prolonged, low-calorie diet. It's the equivalent of the boss walking in and everyone suddenly goes from idly browsing Facebook to being busy and productive. Then, when he's gone, it's back to looking at pictures of cute kittens again!

So first, let's have a quick check to see the boss is around or not. Generally, there are three, big indicators of a low metabolic rate:

1. **Low energy levels:** Has your usual 'get-up-and-go' gone back to bed for a lie-down?
2. **Serious hunger pangs:** Are you so hungry at times that you feel like you could eat your own foot?
3. **Extreme cravings:** Are you so desperate for chocolate, you'd consider selling one of your children for a Kit-Kat?

---

* A client of ours claims his weight issues are due to an overactive chocolate muffin gland. We don't believe him!

There are a few other symptoms: sensitivity to cold, especially in the ends of your fingers and toes, constipation, mood swings and dry skin are also common markers. However, these may be attributable to other issues, not just a low metabolism.

Joking aside, if any of the above symptoms seem familiar, then you either have an undiagnosed medical condition, or you've been dieting too hard or over-training. To be on the safe side, have a chat with your GP or medical practitioner. Then, if everything is okay on the medical front, you're looking at least one month, possibly two for some metabolic rest and recovery.

A bit of metabolic R & R (rest and recovery)

Sorry, but if you've hit a plateau following a long, hard diet, you've got to start eating again. If you're involved in a heavy training programme, especially cardio-type exercise: distance running, etc., then stop completely for a few weeks. We realise that this is probably not what you want to hear but it's a scenario that we frequently deal with. We regularly see clients that train four to five hours per week (often more) and exist on about 1,000 calories day.

If this feels familiar, then you've dug yourself a deep metabolic hole and to carry on digging with further dieting and harder training is not only futile but damaging to your health. Unfortunately, your weight may increase but a lot of it will be water - and only temporary - and then follow our earlier advice about calorie cycling (page 120). It should soon start to fall again and hopefully this time it won't flatline.

Unfortunately, women suffer weight-loss plateaus to a greater degree than men due to the rise and fall of their oestrogen levels. This issue escalates when women start the menopause, causing the body to retain more water and burn less fat.

So, before we move on to some metabolic maintenance solutions, we're going to offer some advice on coping with this issue.

(Note: If you're a man reading this then don't ignore it because men can undergo the 'Male Andropause'. Now, whilst this is nowhere near as severe as the female menopause, it also affects the testosterone/oestrogen balance, causing similar symptoms of fatigue and abdominal weight gain.)

The menopause

This is an extremely tough time for women because their hormonal balance goes completely out of kilter: weight gain is normal and weight loss almost impossible. Ann has been through the menopause twice (yes, it can come back); once in her mid-fifties and again a few years later. Despite all her knowledge, experience, training and general lifestyle, she still gained over 20lbs (about 10kg) the first time and about half as much the second. The lesson she has learnt is, don't fight it by low-calorie dieting, but by exercise and activity.

We've just mentioned the effects on your metabolic rate with low-calorie diets (low thyroid) and when the menopause is over you may be left with a very low metabolic rate. Obviously, this is the very last thing that you need when trying to lose weight. Her advice is to keep training and eating healthily, keep the protein high and carbs low and don't despair (obviously is much easier said than done).

However, it will pass and then some of your weight will drop naturally and the rest you can diet or train off. We'd like to write a lot more about the menopause, but we are stepping into medical territory. Therefore, because we are not medically trained (see the disclaimer at the beginning of the book), we're not too comfortable making anything more than general recommendations for, what is, a very individual and complex problem.

Tip: Ann didn't believe in HRT, but she found that using a bio-identical progesterone cream really helped, especially with hot flushes and many of her clients found it worked for them as well.

Okay, so, what should you be doing to avoid the metabolic mayhem?

Be as neat as possible

NEAT stands for Non-Exercise Activated Thermogenesis. This is when your calorie burning (thermogenesis means 'new heat') increases from sitting around and moves up to light activity, e.g., walking the dog, shopping, gardening, housework, etc. Over the course of a year, NEAT can account for hundreds of thousands of calories. On average, sitting on your bum burns around 60k/cals per hour but just standing burns 90k/cals. A brisk walk burns close to 200k/cals and vigorous housework and gardening up to 300k/cals. (We'll come back to NEAT when we talk about training)

Start resistance training

Try anything: weights, suspension training, resistance bands, circuits, sprints, etc. They are all effective because the more active muscle tissue that you carry, then the higher your metabolic rate. We're not talking about taking up body-building as such but any form of training that will develop lean muscle tissue is great for your metabolism. Cardio training - aerobics, jogging/running, power marching, etc. - is brilliant for health and fitness but it only burns calories whilst you train. Resistance training however, boosts the metabolism for up to 48 hours after the workout. We'll talk about training later and there's tons of help and advice about training on our website.

Reduce stress

Excess stress, both mentally and physically has an enormous, negative impact on your metabolic rate and we'll deal with this critical issue in the next chapter.

Eat more protein

We've already discussed the power of protein and noted many of its benefits. However, it's also highly effective at maintaining your metabolic rate.

Remember, the extra protein in your diet converts to energy, sparing the need for your body to breakdown existing muscle. And as we've just mentioned, less muscle mass equals a lower metabolic rate.

Tip: Unless you have a family history of kidney stones or gout, or a doctor has told you otherwise, then adding a bit more protein to your diet should not cause any issues. We're not talking about binge-eating chicken by the bucket and drinking protein shakes like a steroid-fuelled body-builder, but just try to ensure at least two or three meals per day contain some quality protein.

Okay, so now we've got your metabolism sorted, you need to relax and take it easy.

*****

Chapter 19:
Relax, take it easy

'Feel thinner by making everyone else in your life gain weight'
Anonymous

HOPEFULLY, YOU live in a state of constant bliss, where every traffic light is green, your job is great, and you sleep like a baby. Sadly, in today's, stress-at-every-turn-world, this is doubtful. It's more likely that for you, life is a never-ending traffic jam. At work, you often imagine what your manager would look like without a head and at home, you've the sleep patterns of an insomniac on a caffeine drip. If any of this sounds familiar, then you must act to remedy the situation.

It's vital to understand that chronic stress and lack of sleep will increase belly fat and cause the metabolic rate to back-peddle faster than a politician's pre-election pledges.

So, what's the answer? Well, first let's see how the problem occurs, then we can look at the solutions.

Do battle or run like hell?

We have two, very powerful, stress-responsive hormones designed to keep us alive in times of emergency: cortisol and adrenaline - otherwise known as our fight or flight hormones.

When faced with danger or any perceived threat, adrenaline increases heartrate, makes the muscles contract harder and faster and dilates blood vessels to allow blood to flow quicker. This is all very useful if you need to do battle or run like hell. However, it's cortisol that causes the biggest problems.

Its key role is to make sure that there's sufficient energy available for battling or running by releasing more fat into the bloodstream. Then, to ensure your body's resources keep their focus on staying alive, it temporarily inhibits vital metabolic functions such as digestion, growth, reproduction and your immune system.

So, the primary function of cortisol is to rev up the body for physical activity (which is why we have a surge in cortisol when we wake, to prepare us for the day). But what happens if the stress is purely mental: a broken heart, the commute to work, a big queue at the supermarket, noisy neighbours, etc.? Unfortunately, the answer is the same: increased levels of cortisol and adrenaline.

These hormones evolved in our early history when stress was mainly physical, not mental. This process serves us well when we undergo acute, or short phases of stress, especially physical stress, such as heavy lifting, running for the bus, etc. This is because once the event is over, the body releases stress-busting, feel-good chemicals called endorphins to calm you back down.

The problems develop when you feel as if you exist in a state of perpetual rage that you can't seem to break. One mental stress-event blurs into another, then another, and another until you're walking around like a bear with a bad toothache. But surely, when you are stressed, aren't you burning more energy?

Well, no, not really. In fact, you're more than likely getting fatter, especially around the belly.

How does stress make you fat?

Humans have primary fat cells in the stomach for long-term, emergency use and secondary stores of fat under the skin for more immediate use (which is why your stomach seems to be the last place that shrinks when dieting).

When we become physically or mentally stressed, cortisol stimulates the release of fat from the secondary sites (under the skin) into the bloodstream for more available energy. However, if you don't burn it off, it's reabsorbed by the primary fat cells in your stomach. So, stress makes you shift fat from where it's easy to get at to where it's determined to hang around like a bad smell in a lift.

Long-term (chronic) stress also damages the immune system, reduces the metabolic rate, creates internal inflammation and disrupts the delicate balance of two powerful and important brain chemicals: dopamine and serotonin. This can lead to depression, cravings, comfort eating, and binge-eating. All in all, if you want to lose weight, you don't want chronically-high levels of cortisol in your system.

So, how do you keep them under check?

Stress busters

It's important to find some form of relaxation. This could be anything: reading a book, taking a long bath, meditation, etc., but you need to find a way to turn your brain off for a while. There is a ton of information on the internet about stress release, but we can offer a few helpful ideas:

- ✓ Eating natural, unprocessed foods, especially fibrous veg, will improve digestion and gut health. In turn, this increases the production of a feel-good chemical called serotonin (90% of your serotonin is made in the gut, not the brain).
- ✓ Eating breakfast can help. We already mentioned that breakfast is not necessarily the most important meal of the day, but it counteracts the

natural, morning surge in cortisol. So, as a stress buster, it may be useful.

✓ Take up some vigorous activity or exercise. As we've just mentioned, for thousands of years, mental stress as we know it hardly existed - it was all physical: running, fighting, hunting, etc. This is the reason why post-physical exercise hormones are so potent, they've been in place for years. If you're not already doing so, get off your backside, get some physical exercise done and get these hormones back into the system - your body will love you for it.

✓ Finally, get a good night's sleep. The above points all help towards better sleep, but they mainly deal with the symptoms of existing stress. A good night's sleep 'resets' your stress hormones back to normal levels. It's not difficult to see the downward spiral of daily stress leading to poor sleep, which, in turn increases stress and then poor sleep and more stress and so on and so forth. The problem is often exacerbated by imbibing copious volumes of caffeine during the day to keep you going and a bottle of wine and a Valium sandwich to shut you down in the evening. Numerous sleep studies have shown that a chronic lack of sleep lowers your metabolic rate and increases your appetite, often in as little as four to five days.

Okay, because sleep is such a vital factor in stress management, let's have a look and see if we can improve what happens when you're in the land of nod!

Super sleep

Sleep is very well researched and there's plenty of material online and in bookshops that you may find useful, but generally, the following will help:

✓ No caffeine within 6-8hrs of bedtime.

✓ Abstain from alcohol for a minimum of four evenings per week and try to not drink anything alcoholic within 2-3 hours of bedtime.

✓ Keep the bedroom cool and well ventilated.

✓ Avoid a large meal within 3-4 hours of bedtime.

✓ Computers, phones and tablets emit a specific light frequency that stops the brain from relaxing, so avoid these before bed and if possible, turn off the TV and read a book (a proper one, or at least a black and white Kindle) before retiring.

You can tell from the points above that preparation for sleep is important and what you do within a few hours of bedtime can make all the difference.

Tip: Stress is part and parcel of life. It's inevitable, unavoidable and highly personal because what makes one person tear their hair out, simply washes over another. But if you feel that you're ticking all the right boxes with diet and lifestyle and still struggling to lose weight, look closely at your stress levels and sleeping patterns and you may find the answer to the problem.

Okay, we've talked at length about how your body deals with weight loss, now it's time to learn about the mysterious world of your mind and we'll show you how to sort your head out.

*****

Chapter 20:
The battle starts in your head

'Your body won't go where your mind doesn't push it'
Paul & Ann

WITHOUT DOUBT, the world is full of overweight people who are happy in their life and see no reason to change. They may have the activity levels of a slow-growing fungus and would look at an 'all-you-can-eat-breakfast' as a challenge rather than an option, but everyone has a choice and they've made theirs.

On the flip-side however, there are millions of men, women and children who struggle with their weight and are unhappy about it - often desperately so. Despite their best efforts, nothing seems to work. In general, this is not necessarily their fault because they keep trying unsuitable diets that don't suit their lifestyle. Not to mention that much of the information found in the popular media is simply myth, urban legend or a magic trick of some sort (usually involving the latest dodgy supplement or fad diet).

But why won't it happen? 'What's wrong?', you may ask. Well, here is where we need to clarify the difference between what you want your body to do and what it can do. Because they are often far from the same.

Sort your head out

One of the fundamental concepts involved in both losing weight, and possibly more importantly, keeping it off, is realising that it's an ongoing and never-ending, lifelong civil war that rages within yourself. Your head - driven by emotion - wants you to lose weight, but your body, forged by human evolution and its fantastic survival instinct will rally its defences and fight back against any attempt to reduce its precious, life-saving fat stores.

At a subconscious level your body recognises this. Your cells, tissues and organs know more about biology, genetics and physics than a boat-load of Oxford science professors, with Stephen Hawking as captain. Whilst your body understands the rules of engagement in this eternal civil war, your head, at a conscious level, doesn't.

For example, you may think that you can shed lots of fat very quickly but sadly, your body won't let you because it has some specific limitations. Such as:

- ✓ Fat cannot burn without the presence of oxygen - it's purely an aerobic system. This means that the amount of oxygen you can get into your system is a limiting factor. To give you an idea, Tour de France cyclists - possibly the fittest people on the planet - can only metabolise about 400-500 calories of fat per hour. For a normal person, then, unless you can develop the ability to breathe through your ears, you're not even going to get close.
- ✓ You can't sweat fat out. If you could, you'd end up looking like a 19th century English Channel swimmer who's covered in lard to protect against the chilly water. Could you imagine the smell of warm fat oozing out of your pores on a sweltering day?
- ✓ It won't just melt either. If it did, where would it go? It can't pass through your kidneys, and your intestines only bring stuff in, they can't take it out. So, if you don't burn it off, it just comes back as fat.
- ✓ Finally, and the biggest issue of all, you can't create more energy without creating more heat (Laws of thermodynamics). In fact, if you

could burn fat at the levels necessary to make an immediate, noticeable difference you would become so hot your ear wax would melt and your hair catch fire. Flippancy aside, there have been many fatalities in the UK due to taking an illegal fat burning compound called DNP. In each case, the coroner reported that death occurred because individual's organs had been 'cooked' due to a massive increase in body temperature. This is a crucial point to understand because if your 'fat-burning' pill or programme worked as well as it claims, then you would notice it. Your heart would be pumping, and you'd be sweating because of the extra heat produced from burning more fat. Now, we're not saying that there is no effect at all, because you could possibly burn a further 300-500 calories over a 24-hour period and not really notice it, but it won't be in the thousands of calories.

So, it doesn't matter if your auntie Geraldine overheard her hairdresser talking about a neighbour whose best friend lost half her body weight in two days on the same diet that the actress from Eastenders is on - it's not going to happen.

But why is this, because it seems very unfair? Well, it's got a lot to do with your ancestors.

*****

Chapter 21:
Don't blame your genes

'Genetics only loads the gun. It's lifestyle that pulls the trigger!'
Anonymous

Genetically speaking you are the end-product of an ancestry that spans hundreds of thousands of years. Therefore, you have a genetic makeup that is both energy efficient and has the capacity to store a bit of extra fat for times of need. How do we know? Because if you didn't, you wouldn't be here.

Your early forbears survived conditions that would make the selection process for the SAS look like a picnic in the park with some ginger beer. Now, everyone knows the SAS are tough. They storm enemy encampments armed with little more than night-vision goggles and a rolled-up newspaper! Plus, they can live for months on nettles, toothpaste and rainwater. They are the embodiment of human resolve, yet you share the same genes. Fundamentally, there is little or no difference between you that any type of genetic testing could identify. However, don't go storming any random Middle-Eastern embassy just yet because there's some work to do first.

Get your hand out of the biscuit tin

Throughout our long history, survival has usually involved being faster and smarter than your next meal.

In fact, to our ancestors, 'fast food' was usually their next meal disappearing at speed over the hill!

Yet, in our 'modern' civilised society food has more to do with pleasure, not survival.

In fact, the only hunting for food we do nowadays is rummaging through the biscuit barrel to find the last chocolate digestive.

For most of the western world, 'survival' is only a few feet away in the fridge, five minutes by car to the supermarket or, God forbid if that's too much effort, a couple of clicks on your computer. You must understand that every device in your house that saves time and energy also saves calories as well!

Tip: Recreate the type of foraging diet that would mimic the calorie burning of our ancestors' hunter-gatherer lifestyle. Simply hide your partner's packed-lunch just before they set off for work. Just a thought!

Is it your fault or not?

Our evolution and genetics have now created a modern-day paradox. Biologically-speaking, your weight issues are not entirely your fault, i.e., you have inherited, not created, your energy-efficient, fat-gaining genes. However, mentally-speaking, it is your fault if you've merely sat on your bum all day with your hand stuck firmly inside the family-sized pack of Doritos and Domino's pizza on permanent redial.

Help is at hand

To help resolve this very personal issue, we try to help our clients to accept four, basic principles:

1. Your genetics have only loaded the gun, it's you that's pulled the trigger.
2. If you're healthy, capable of movement and making your own decisions, then it's your choice and yours alone.
3. If you want something badly enough, you'll find a way; if you don't, you'll find an excuse.
4. The time for excuses is over.

Now, at this point, you may feel as if your problems are insurmountable; that there is an enormous mountain to climb. But helping you to overcome your issues is what we're here for and this final part of the book is all about planning your journey and making the route as easy as possible.

So, what's the next step? Well, let's have a look and see if we can make life a little easier by setting off on the right path. For that, we need to change your mind about how you view the weight-loss world. Let's see you how to keep the same old you but make it better.

*****

Chapter 22:
You, but better

'If you want something bad enough, you'll find a way.
If you don't you'll find an excuse'
Anonymous

THERE ARE many obvious reasons why people want to lose weight: holidays, weddings, health issues, etc. However, there is a deeper, underlying reason driving the decision, something called a Positive Change. This is when you decide to make a fundamental change to your life that you perceive will make you a happier, better person. And this is a good thing. However, if you set off down the wrong path, you can quickly turn a positive change into a negative experience, which is not so good. Let's see how to keep things on track.

Set realistic goals

Getting a svelte bikini body, or a ripped six-pack is one thing but keeping it is another problem entirely. Sorry, but the sacrifices you'll have to make to lose so much weight won't suddenly stop when you hit your targets. In fact, they may even get worse! You may currently be a size 18 and you'd love to be a size 10 but your life may be more fun as a size 12, or a six-pack would be nice, but a flat stomach is much easier to maintain.

Your weight is irrelevant.

Your weight is only relevant if you partake in a sport that has specific weight categories, e.g., boxing. The true gauge is what the tape measure says, how your clothes fit and how you feel. We don't say this lightly, as we've seen too many eating disorders, body dysmorphic conditions and awful levels of self-loathing from an obsessive fixation on weight targets.

Another reason to stop weighing yourself is that it's all too easy to think that all weight loss is equal. That every pound off the scales is a good pound. But what if you're only losing water, or even worse, muscle tissue? How do you think you would look if you lost all your muscle mass but kept the fat? Is that look you want: soft and flabby? Or would you rather look sleek and toned? Again, the scales won't tell you but your clothes or the tape measure will.

Tip: To gauge progress properly, first find some clothes that are slightly too tight. Then, your next target is not what you weigh but how these clothes fit. Finally, when they're comfy, find some more that are just a little tight and keep repeating until you are where you want to be.

Ditch the scales

Checking your weight is one thing but if the result directly impacts your mood and what you eat for the day, then there may be an underlying problem. For example:

- ✓ Are you anxious before you step on the scales?
- ✓ Are you extra happy for the rest of day if you've lost weight or depressed if you haven't?
- ✓ If you've not lost anything do you decide to either not eat for the rest of the day or change what you had planned to something with fewer calories?
- ✓ Do you weigh yourself twice a day?
- ✓ Do you empty your bladder and bowels first?
- ✓ Do you know your weight to the decimal point?

If you answer, 'yes' to any of these questions, then it's likely that your relationship with the scales is already unhealthy and we strongly recommend that you put the scales away for a while.

Tip: If you can't live without your bathroom scales, then only weigh yourself two or three times per week and work on the averages for the week, not the specifics. And tell yourself that that you'll make any necessary changes the following week, not today.

Don't confuse fat weight with water weight

The main constituent of a human being is water. About sixty percent of you is nothing more than the wet stuff that falls out of the sky. The reason we mention this is that when you first start a diet, especially a diet that involves dropping carbs, water is the main thing that you lose.

On average, carbs (sugars and starches) make your body hold between 4-7lbs (about 2-3kg) of extra water and usually add in a further 2-3lbs (1-2kg) of intestinal bulk as they pass through your system.

So, you can see how easy it would be to quickly drop 7-10lbs (about 4-5kg) by dropping carbs out of your diet. Yet, it's only intestinal bulk and water that's disappeared, not fat. So, the first few pounds lost on a crash diet is nothing more than a long wee and a big poo (too much information?).

Likewise, the reverse happens with rapid weight gain when you come off a low carb diet plan. Again, it's water that's come back, not fat. Also, the flow and ebb of various hormones, such as oestrogen or testosterone affect how your body retains or releases water. So, at various times of the month, you may be heavier or lighter, but again, it's water, not fat.

Tip: For a man to move his belt notch by an inch or a woman to drop a dress-size, it would take a calorie deficit (or surplus if the weight is going the other way) of tens of thousands of calories. Therefore, any sudden, overnight shift of one or two pounds (approx. 0.5-1kg) can only be water – it cannot be fat!

Work on your willpower

Sorry, but we can't claim our methods are going to be a 'willpower-free zone', because you will have to assume some responsibility for your actions. We've already mentioned that you can't have your cake and eat it but here's a few tips that may allow you the occasional slice:

- ✓ It's unlikely that a diamond-hard willpower will simply appear overnight. So, don't expect a visit from the 'willpower fairy' and suddenly, all your problems are solved. Yes, going 'cold-turkey' works for some but a gradual shift is often the best way. Willpower takes time, effort and practice to develop.
- ✓ Whenever possible, plan your day and take food with you. This could be a lunch for work or even some healthy snacks if you're just out and about. Also, you'll usually find your willpower cowering behind the sofa when you're stressed or hungry; so again, avoid the situation and be prepared.
- ✓ Work on creating new, 'positive' habits. Habitual and regular decisions require less willpower than having to make new choices.
- ✓ Exert your willpower selectively, particularly at the supermarket. Imagine, for example, that every day you eat three chocolate digestive biscuits with your afternoon coffee. To save calories, you take the decision to cut back to just one. You now face yet another daily willpower decision, as every afternoon you will have to exert your willpower to stop eating your usual three biscuits. An easier option would be to make one 'willpower' choice at the time of purchase and buy plain biscuits instead (which have fewer calories). You can still have three biscuits and reduce your calorie intake at the same time.

Enjoy the journey

It's easy to tie yourself in knots worrying about all the things you can't do when trying to lose weight. It can all become a bit 'negative'.

Yet this needn't be so. Congratulate yourself on every step forward as the dress sizes come down and the belt tightens and be happy about what you've achieved, not miserable about what you haven't done yet. We all know time flies, so recall an event last year: wedding, birthday, holiday, etc, and think how fast the time has gone. Then, either compare your progress to that point in time or think if you'd started your weight-loss plan then, how good you'd look now and then project that thought to another event in a few months.

Keeping positive is important and don't forget how far you've come. Remember that the objective of undertaking a positive change is a happier life, not an unhappy one.

Be consistent

Stop trying to get everything right, just start getting it right more often than getting it wrong. In the long run, consistency will beat perfection hands down every time. Simply because life is never straight forward, and it rarely, if ever, goes to plan. There will be times when you can stick to a great eating plan and times when you can't. Small weight fluctuations are both inevitable and natural, so accept it – just don't let it get out of hand.

Tip: Live by the 80/20 principle: 80% of the foods you eat and the life you lead will take you a step forward on the road to success, whilst allowing a 20% detour down the naughty path to keep you sane.

Finally, put your health first

The most important positive change you can make is to be healthier because bikini bodies and six-packs simply pale into insignificance when compared to your health.

It's been said that 'nothing tastes as good as skinny feels', but we'd argue that nothing tastes as bad as hospital food! There's no point in 'looking good' if it makes you ill. Especially while you watch the quality of your life spiral incessantly downwards as the list of all the things you can't do, or eat, gets longer and longer as your diet gets harder. If you pin 'health first' to the top of your 'to-do' list and change your diet and lifestyle accordingly, then weight loss will follow.

We can't stress this point strongly enough. **Almost every success story we've had over the years, where the weight comes off and stays off, has begun with changing to a healthier lifestyle. One that involves eating better, cutting back on the junk where possible and increasing activity levels. Aim for this, and weight loss always happens.**

Remember, we're not talking about being a perfect version of you, just the same old you, but better.

******

PART 2:
TRAIN SMARTER, NOT HARDER

'All exercise comes at a cost. But that doesn't necessarily mean it always comes with a benefit'
Paul & Ann

Chapter 23:
Exercise - it's all a bit confusing!

'We can't reinvent the wheel, but we can make sure
you've got the right set of Tyres!'
Paul & Ann

THE WORLD OF exercise science is so vast it borders on infinite. Facts, figures, statistics, conclusions, proclamations and opinions travel the world at light-speed and are now instantly available at the click of a mouse. There is so much information - but not necessarily knowledge - available in print, apps and on the Internet that it's difficult to know where to start.

Type 'fitness' into an Amazon book search and you'll get over 170,000 titles (weight loss/diet has nearly 60,000) and YouTube will provide nearly six million videos (now that's what we would call binge-watching). So, it's no wonder it's all a bit baffling as to what you should do for the best.

It's very possible that this plethora of data, facts, figures and opinions is the reason why Britons wasted over £45 million on gym memberships[10] in 2015 and why the current weight loss/diet industry in the UK is worth almost £10 billion - everyone has an opinion, but no one seems to have the ultimate answer. Best-selling author, Richard Paul Evans sums it up nicely when he says that, "we are swimming in an ocean of knowledge, yet drowning in ignorance".

It's not just the diet and exercise industry that receives millions either.

The annual turnover of sports clothing and footwear giants Nike in 2017 was $35billion[11]. To us, these unbelievable amounts of money that are thrown around are an obvious indicator that the 'eat less, move more' dictum is not as simple as it sounds. If it was, the world would be full of very fit, very thin people instead of the estimated 1.5 billion[12] overweight individuals that walk (or plod?) the Earth today (but looking at Nike's turnover, at least they're wearing nice trainers!).

Train smarter, not harder

So, with all this uncertainty abound in the industry that we've spent pretty much all our lives in so far, we're going to try and explain as much as possible about the rules of exercise and training.

We're going to do our very best to put nearly seventy years of combined experience into this book - all under the 'some important stuff you really need to know' tagline. We're not going to tell you that our system is the last word in exercise science. Or that it will show you the ultimate work-out and replace your unwanted wobbly bits with rock-hard muscle within just six weeks.

No, we're happy to leave that particular type of noxious drivel to the popular media.

If you've read any of our other work, you will have realised that we don't claim to be miracle workers. Sad to say that there is often no simple answer to life's problems. Much of what you eventually undertake will have to be tried, tested and evaluated by you as an individual. Why? Because, like many things in life, what works for one person will not work as well for another. It helps, however, if you have a solid foundation to start from.

The most bang for your buck!

Despite spending most of our adult lives in and around the gym, neither of us has ever wanted to waste our time and effort when working out. So, we set about reducing every workout to its bare minimum. As with our dietary advice, we work on the basis that it's not how much we need to do but how little! The general idea was to get from each workout what the Americans would call 'the most bang for your buck!'

Eventually, we worked out, what we thought were very simple guidelines: basic rules that once learnt, could easily be applied to whatever exercise protocol you were following. Therefore, improving its efficacy in both time and results. It wouldn't matter if you were body building or marathon running, the rules would be the same.

However, we have neither the space nor time to cover every single possible workout protocol that we know. We could, and hopefully will, at some point write entire volumes and books about the specific routines regarding weight training, body building, fitness and strength conditioning, boxing, martial arts, etc., (and you can find some training videos on our website).

KISS: keep it simple stupid

This book is all about covering the very basic, fundamental ideas and concepts behind exercise. However, we'll not leave you totally empty-handed and we will touch on a few simple workouts. It's only taken us half a lifetime to figure out, so hopefully, you should be able to avoid many of the pitfalls we fell into and subsequently, you won't waste as much time deciding what suits you best.

In the next few chapters we'll explain some of the terminologies that you'll need to understand if you want to design your own workouts and routines.

Rather than throw everything at you in one big (tedious?) lump, each chapter will explain a few important and necessary terminology.

Then, the next one will take it a step further and so on, building layer upon layer of information until we've covered as much as possible. Along the way, we'll talk about workload and effort and clarify the true effects of fat-burning routines.

We'll explain the differences between aerobic, anaerobic, cardio-vascular and resistance type training and finally show you the 'nuts and bolts' of an effective programme that can be adapted to suit your requirements.

To cater for as many readers as possible, we've cut back on the science as much as possible but hopefully retained a fair amount of technical data to paint a comprehensive picture of exercise methodology. If you find any part of the book difficult to follow (or just generally boring), then just look for the summaries scattered around the text, which should keep you abreast of the information.

 Note: We will also continually use the word 'athlete' as a generic term when explaining the effects of exercise on an individual. To make matters clear, we consider an 'athlete' to be anyone that undertakes any form of specific activity or exercise regime. We're not talking about Usain Bolt or any other similar top-class competitive Olympian but about you, the reader. To us, as soon as you put your trainers on and hit the gym, fitness class, bicycle, treadmill or whatever, you are an athlete. Also, for the purposes of simplicity, most of the examples we'll use will involve running or power-marching.

This is primarily because pretty much everyone can easily identify with these activities. Whereas specific exercises, such as the 'bench press' or 'deadlift' in weight training, may not be to everyone's 'cup of tea' and therefore, the ideas we are trying to get across may be lost.

So, first things first, and in the spirit of the 'Marshmallow Diet' (i.e. we're going to poke a bit of fun at it) let's have a look at The Celebrity Workout.

*****

Chapter 24:
The celebrity workout

'The 'Hollywood' six pack: 75% hard work 25% airbrush?'
Paul & Ann

THE CELEBRITY workout is very simple. First become famous for something or other (talent is not always a given). Next, employ a chef, personal assistant, live-in nanny, manager, chauffeur and optional Feng Shui expert to remove all the 'negative energy' in your life (and about five-grand from your wallet). This is necessary to take care of all the mundane aspects of your life, leaving you two to three hours of free time per day to devote to exercise.

Alternatively, go on a 'Strictly Come and Get Me off this X-Factoring Ice Rink' reality show and once again, spend most of the day jumping up and down (falling over is not actually necessary but makes good TV) and running about a lot and surprise, surprise, you'll lose two stone. Note: A good sob story, a few tears and regularly repeating "I'm doing it for my Nan" may be required, but sadly, this will not increase fat loss!

Getting in shape can be a full-time occupation

Remember when Daniel Craig walked out of the sea in his role as the new James Bond in Casino Royale, with abs and muscles all over the place, looking fantastic.

Well, just after the film was released, we were in a pub one weekend when we were recognised by an overweight, middle-aged bloke who used to 'train' at the same gym we did a few years earlier (we use the term loosely – he spent more time talking than training). He wanted to know why, after many years of going to the gym, he didn't look anywhere near as good.

The answer was simple: Daniel Craig didn't drink twenty pints of beer per week, nor did he eat burgers, kebabs or any other rubbish and he trained a damn sight more often than two hours per week. **In fact, in the few months prior to filming, he was probably busting a gut in the gym 1-2 hours per day, 6 days per week!** For professional actors, getting in shape for a role can be a full-time occupation.

The guy wondered if it was possible for him to get into such good shape in just a few weeks. "Easy", we replied: "Just pack in your job for the next ten weeks and employ us as your full-time trainers and nutritionists. We will virtually move in with you and take over your life, taking control of everything you eat and drink and training you an average of three to four hours per day. We will clear all the crap out of your fridge and kitchen cupboards, replacing it with water, chicken, salmon, eggs, broccoli and spinach.

We will be at your door at 5.30 am for a 45-minute morning run, then it's a healthy porridge and chai seed breakfast followed a little later by some weight training for an hour. You can have a light tuna salad for lunch, a little snooze, then fitness and stamina training or boxing for a couple of hours. You then go home for dry chicken or steamed fish with low carbs for dinner and finally an early night because you're doing it all over again the next day and you need to get some rest.

You will get up when we say, eat and drink what we tell you and go to bed when we say - in other words, you will do everything we demand.

You won't be able to work because you won't have time as you'll be too busy either training or sleeping. And don't even think about drinking any alcohol or eating any pastries; it's just high protein and low carb veggies for you until we see those abs on display. Strangely, he declined our offer.

Yet, this is not fantasy, it's how film stars like Will Smith, Demi Moore, Hugh Jackman, etc. get in shape for their roles.

A year's-worth of training in a few months

Celebrities are only human, and their bodies obey the same laws of physics and biology as everyone else, but they have access to facilities that mere mortals such as us can only dream of. This is not to say they don't work hard to achieve their fantastic physiques because they undoubtedly do. It's just not a level playing field comparing them to the ordinary public who have no option other than work 9am-5pm all year, sort the kids out, prepare meals, do the laundry and ironing, go to the supermarket, walk the dog, etc. etc. - in other words, real life!

We're not suggesting that you'll never look like a 'celeb', because it most certainly is achievable - it's just not going to happen as quick. What a 'celeb' can look like in just twelve weeks may take you twelve months but it can be done if you try hard enough and devote time, effort, and above all, consistency to your training and nutrition.

There are countless examples of TV & film stars whose bodyweight seems to go up and down like a yo-yo on amphetamines. They often admit to starving themselves to get in shape for their DVDs. Then find themselves unable to maintain the strict 'two-hour' daily workouts once the publicity and promo-work has passed. Therefore, it's very, very important to set realistic targets, because exercise and good nutrition must become a way of life, not just an occasional hobby.

So, in the next chapter, we'll start right at the beginning and cover some Basic Training Principles.

*****

Chapter 25:
Training: the basic principles

*'Training is hard, excuses are easy. Unfortunately, excuses
don't burn calories'.*
Anonymous

EXERCISE SCIENCE can be a complicated business, with intricate equations and impressive terminology used to determine angles of movement, degrees of force, maximal power output, etc. But, to the average person trying to get a bit fitter or lose some weight, it's mostly a load of indecipherable, irrelevant old tosh! To make it worse, it's also really confusing.

Most people who decide to take up some form of exercise/activity, particularly for weight loss, will give up within the first month, mainly for the following reasons:

1. **Their expectation of the amount of fat they hope to lose is too high. Unfortunately, when it comes to how fast we can burn fat during exercise, humans must make do with the replacement bus service, not the high-speed train.**
2. **They don't know how to put an effective exercise programme together.**

This problem is often exacerbated at the same time with a drastic reduction in calorie intake (usually as the result of post-alcohol-fuelled New Year's resolutions).

It can be hard enough just asking your body to start doing some physically demanding work, possibly for the first time in years, without starving it as well. The blend of tough workouts, minimal food and no real idea of what you're doing is a recipe for unmitigated failure.

Understanding the basic principles of exercise is not difficult but it is absolutely vital that you try and grasp them. Otherwise, at best you'll be working much harder than you need to, and at worst, you'll end up packing in training because you'll see little or no progress.

Tip: We generally suggest to our clients that their New Year's resolutions start in January with a good exercise programme and a 'clean-up' of their diet, i.e. cut out all the crap. But don't think about drastically cutting calories until Spring, when the days get longer, and the weather feels better. Attempting a tough diet in the middle of a cold, dark winter, when all your body wants is lovely warm comfort food, is definitely in the 'Top 10 mistakes to make when dieting'.

Stress forces change

Despite a general aversion to being stressed, it's the primary cause that forces our body to make changes and modifications. The constant worry of survival, food, sex, illness, death, etc. is the one constant of every living creature on Earth. The ability to adapt to the demands of stress, either physical or mental, is the driving force behind our evolution.

This very simple but essential physiological process provides our fundamental principle: **Stress + Recovery = Modification**

Let's explain this a little further.

1. **Stress**: The demand or load placed on the muscles, heart and lungs. When the body is placed under some form of physical stress that it struggles to cope with, tiny amounts of damage (micro-tears) are created within the tissues that are being worked. This damage is

subsequently repaired in such a way as to be able to cope better the next the same stress is applied. For example, for an average person, running a marathon would place a greater stress on the body than jogging round the park.

2. **Recovery**: A period of rest and recuperation before the next workout, where the damage is being repaired. This is not just time but also includes the amount of both food and sleep.

3. **Modification**: The subsequent repair work and adjustments your body makes to be able to deal more efficiently with the demands it's placed under. This can be improvements in cardiovascular fitness, muscle tone, strength, etc.

These processes must occur in the above order: you cannot go from stress to modification without going through recovery first.

Also, all three must also be in relative proportion. For example, too much stress with insufficient recovery would limit modification as the body is constantly in a state of repair. Likewise, if there is insufficient load on the body (stress), then recovery is not necessary and there is no need to make any modifications.

Summary:

- ✓ **Your body will not make any changes unless it's forced to.**
- ✓ **Any modifications are both proportionate and relative to the demands that it's placed under. For example, running won't make you better at lifting weights and vice versa.**

The next stage

Let's take the basic principle of **Stress + Recovery = Modification** a stage further and cover three more concepts which will help you to choose what types of exercise will suit your goals.

These are:

1. **Work**: the type of exercise or activity you undertake: weights, badminton, running a 5k, playing football, etc
2. **Time**: how long you spend on the activity
3. **Intensity**: how much effort you put into the activity

To explain how this works, let's take an example of a 5k (approx. 3 miles) run. To complete the distance, you could either:

a) Stroll (2 miles per hour)
b) Power-march (4 mph)
c) Jog (6 mph)
d) Run like the clappers (12 mph)

In each case the work is the same, i.e. covering a 5k distance but the intensity varies from an easy stroll (2mph) up to a torturous sprint (12mph). The time taken to complete the distance would reduce at the same rate that the effort and intensity increases: an easy stroll for 90 minutes; a steady power-march for 45 minutes; a fairly tough jog for 30 minutes or a spleen-busting run for about 15 minutes.

But how are these terms relevant to you? Well, these terms allow us to consider the following:

✓ Calorie expenditure during the workout.
✓ Increased Calorie expenditure (higher metabolic rate) after the workout. This process is called EPOC (Exercise Post Oxygen Consumption) and we'll come to this shortly.

Strangely, in the 5k scenario, all the options: A, B, C & D will have about the same energy expenditure during the workout. This may sound slightly ludicrous at first but let us explain because it's all about that essential, but rarely thought of element: oxygen.

Oxygen: life, death and fat-burning

Despite what the makers of dodgy pills and wonder fat-busting workouts may claim, human energy expenditure has one, major limiting factor: oxygen consumption.

Without oxygen we can only burn fuel for a few seconds. In fact, we can't even burn body fat at all without oxygen (we burn sugar if oxygen isn't available). Therefore, almost all our energy expenditure – especially burning fat – only occurs when we can get enough oxygen to the working muscles.

In humans, this works out at about 5k/cals of energy for every litre of oxygen we metabolise. So, assuming you have a healthy set of lungs, then the more out of breath you are, the more calories you burn. (We'll come back to this vital point in Chapter 24: The best fat-burning workouts.)

So, back to the 5k scenario, you would take about the same total number of breaths by breathing heavily for 15 minutes as breathing lightly for 90minutes, therefore, calorie expenditure is about the same.

Note: an 'average' 168lb (76kg) male would burn 336 calories whilst walking for 90 minutes and 330 calories for running at 12mph for 15 minutes.

After the event

But what happens to your metabolic rate after you completed your 5k? In options A & B (stroll/power-march) it will return to normal almost immediately. In option C (jogging), it may be elevated slightly for a couple of hours. But with option D (all-out sprint), it's likely to stay high for 12-24 hours, possibly longer. It's been well proven that intense exercise of any sort (especially weight training) elevates your metabolism for a substantial period after you've trained. This effect is commonly referred to as EPOC - Excess Post-Exercise Oxygen Consumption.

But don't get too excited just yet because depending upon age, gender, muscle mass, etc., it could be as little as an extra one hundred calories over the 12-48-hour, post-workout period. The science behind this effect is highly debateable. Some studies claim it's a paltry amount - 50-150 calories or so - whilst other research makes claims that just 3-5 minutes of intense exercise, twice per week, will rev up your metabolic rate so high you will have a beach-fit bikini body in a fortnight.

Our experience would lean towards the lower amount, simply because if your metabolism was on fire to this obviously exaggerated degree, then you would be as well! As your metabolic rate goes up, so does your heart rate, oxygen consumption and body temperature. Now, whilst this does happen, the overall amount is not substantial enough to account for thousands of calories.

We'll explain in later chapters about how evolution has shaped our lives, but it's worth a quick mention here. Humans didn't evolve sitting around all day playing video games and watching telly. If we had, we'd have an enormous, well-cushioned bum that didn't go numb after sitting for a couple of hours (or is that just us?). Also, we are superbly designed for high levels of activity. Indeed, many of our essential rest and recovery, stress-busting hormones won't even bother getting out of bed unless we're physically working hard and building up a good sweat.

Tip: The extra calories burnt during the post-exercise period following intense exercise may only be small but the effect on your hormonal balance however, is definitely big. Mood and sleep patterns improve, stress levels drop, muscles become sensitive to insulin (we deal with carbs more effectively), etc. It's as if your body has stepped up into the next gear and runs more smoothly.

Why not just get your gym kit on and go for it?

So, is the answer to your workout problems to simply jump in at the deep end and train so hard you pass out at the end of every training session? The straight answer is no, definitely not!

In fact, this would have the opposite effect of solving your problems because the amount of stress from training consistently at such high intensities would completely overwhelm your body's ability to recover and you would go backwards, rather than forwards.

Remember that demand, recovery and modification have, not only to be in the correct balance, but also in this order:

- ✓ Stress - (demand) followed by -
- ✓ Recovery - (rest, food and sleep) and finally -
- ✓ Modification - (improved fitness, tone, strength, health, etc.)

We've already noted this but it's worth mentioning again. You cannot adapt to any type of exercise without first going through a recovery phase. It's not just the muscles that are affected but both your central nervous system and your immune system are temporarily stressed as well.

So, if you are continuously putting your body under highly demanding workouts, not only will you not make the progress you seek, but it's very likely that you will make yourself mentally and physically ill as well.

Variety is vital

Generally, all exercise programmes, regardless of type - weights, boxing, cardio-vascular/fitness, aerobics, etc., have pros and cons. But you should strive to incorporate a broad range of intensities from low or moderate levels right through to working hard enough to drip with sweat.

This maximises cardiovascular development, strength, recovery, and most important for weight/fat loss, burns calories. In the next chapter, we're going to go into more detail about how to determine just the right amount of balance between work, time and intensity. But for now, we'd just mention a common saying in the world of exercise: **you can train long, or you can train hard, but you can't train long and hard.**

Summary

✓ The harder you breathe, the more calories you burn.

✓ Exercise that makes you breathless may elevate your metabolism for up to 48 hours afterwards. Whilst this may only be a few hundred calories at most, it will build up to a substantial amount over the forthcoming weeks and months.

✓ All programmes should contain a variety of exercises (work), as well as how long you do them for (time) and how much effort you put into them (intensity).

A 'neat' way to burn extra calories

We've noted this earlier, but we'll cover it now in a little more detail. A specific exercise programme is not the only way to raise your metabolic rate because there is another NEAT way to burn extra some extra calories (this doesn't mean tidying the gym after your workout). NEAT is an acronym for Non-Exercise Activated Thermogenesis (thermogenesis is a fancy name for energy expenditure).

Very simply, NEAT is the extra amount of energy you burn when you're more active than just watching telly or reading a book, but less active than participating in a specific sport or exercise-based activity. It covers such things as household chores, gardening, shopping, walking about, climbing stairs, etc.

Let's give you a terrifying statistic: It's not uncommon for the average British citizen to spend over 80% of their week either lying or sitting down.

Now, we're not big believers in the absolute accuracy of any form of calorie expenditure calculators. But purely for the sake of comparison, the table on the next page should give you a rough idea of how many calories you'd burn per hour when undertaking a range of non-exercise type activities.

Activity (60 minutes)	Weight: 12st (168lbs/76kg)	Weight :14st (196lbs/89kg)	Weight: 16st (224lbs/101kg)
Lying down or sitting quietly	101	118	134
Sitting – office work	128	149	170
Standing – office/retail	165	192	220
Housework	286	333	381
Gardening (general)	269	314	358
Walking 3mph (4.8kph) steady pace	336	392	448

(If you would like to determine your own amounts, visit www.calorielab.com/burned/)

This demonstrates how easy it is to increase your daily energy expenditure by just being a bit more active, especially being on your feet for longer periods of time. You can see quite clearly that walking at a steady pace burns about three times the amount of sitting down or just generally being inactive.

Simple NEAT options

Simple options to increase your activity levels, without undertaking a specific exercise regime include:

- ✓ Regularly walking to and/or from work.
- ✓ If that's not possible, you could get on the bus 2 - 3 stops further away than normal and then get off 2-3 stops early.
- ✓ If you drive, you could park your car further away from your place of work.
- ✓ Go for a walk during your lunch break.
- ✓ Take the stairs instead of the lift or escalator.

Whilst each bit of NEAT may only account for a few hundred extra calories per week, the cumulative effect over a period of time is astonishing. Add in a good diet and a bit of exercise and you'll find you hit your targets much quicker than you first thought.

The other brilliant trick about NEAT is how it (along with a good exercise programme) will keep the weight off once you've achieved your weight/fat loss goals.

Tip: If you want to burn a few more calories and improve your fitness without leaving your home, you can try what we call 'Soap Training'. Get hold of an exercise bike or cross-trainer and when your favourite soap-opera is on, jump on and pedal away at a nice steady pace. Then, for the next 30 minutes or so while you watch the latest births, deaths, brawls, affairs, murders and other catastrophes (the entire A-Z of humanity in a half-hour episode) which blast out on a nightly basis from the goggle-box, you can still burn off some fat.

*****

Chapter 26:
Making good progress

'Would you rather be covered in sweat at the gym or covered in clothes on the beach?'
Anonymous

NO ONE IS born fit. Some have a natural propensity to becoming athletic whilst it's a struggle for others. But everyone has a common denominator: they all started at the beginning and worked their way up to whatever standard they are now.

The universal system they'll have used is called Progressive Overload. Each month, week or training session, an athlete of any standard will try and improve their fitness, strength, stamina, skills, etc. by gradually increasing either, how long they train for, or how much effort they put in. In other words, they keep increasing the demands their body must cope with.

For example, if your target is to run a 5k race (about 3 miles) for charity but walking up a flight of stairs makes you wheeze like a pensioner with a life-long 60-a-day smoking habit, then trying to do 5k on your first attempt would probably put you in the hospital.

The way to train for a 5k would be to break the distance down into more manageable chunks. Start off with a 2k target and on day one, run for a short while until you tire and then walk a bit. When you've recovered slightly, run a little more until you feel the need to walk again. Keep at this alternating run/walk pace until you've covered your first target of 2k

Initially, your legs will be sore, so let them recover for a few days and then try again. Over the next few sessions things won't seem quite as hard, and you find you can run a little further before you need to walk again. Keep repeating this until you can run 2k without walking (or using your inhaler). Then, using the same run/walk method, raise the distance to 3k, then 4k, until finally, you can run the entire 5k distance.

Sun tan or sun burn?

One of the easiest ways of understanding the concept of progressive overload is to use the analogy of getting a suntan (wow - fat loss, fitness and a tan - all in one chapter!).

Without doubt, suntans are best developed gradually. As opposed to just standing under the blaze of a hot Sun without any sun screen protection for hours on the first day of your holiday. Done properly, slightly increasing your skin's exposure to the Sun by a little more each day is the best way to get healthy tan; otherwise you end up burning rather than tanning.

How does getting a tan relate to exercise? Well, the method by which your body acclimatises to the Sun's rays is precisely the same system that makes your body adapt to exercise: it uses a finely-honed self-defence mechanism designed to combat stress.

With the Sun, your skin can't cope with the damaging ultraviolet (UV) light, the stress of which overloads the skin's natural defences against sunlight. So, to protect itself, your skin darkens, because dark skin absorbs less UV light than light skin. In the case of exercise, your heart, lungs, muscles, bones, joints, etc. can become damaged by being 'overloaded' with the demands they're placed under. Subsequently, they also protect themselves by making specific changes in their structure that allows them to be able to perform the extra work without being damaged again. So, in the same way that your tanned skin can now tolerate the Sun's rays, your muscles, etc. can withstand the effects of exercise-induced stress.

In both cases, the relevant word is 'overload'. For the body to adapt, there first must be some form of high demand or overload, without which, nothing happens. However, if there's too much, then the resultant damage is greater than the body's defence mechanisms can cope with. In the case of the Sun, you can end up with burn instead of a tan. With exercise, the muscles and tendons can either completely tear or become so sore, you can't even walk properly, let alone do any further exercise for days afterwards.

Going back to the 5k run, in the same way your skin builds a resistance to the sun, your legs have now built a resistance to running by breaking the stress down into manageable chunks. Each one slightly harder than the last and you have now successfully completed your first 5k via the very simple system of progressive overload. The same method would apply to any type of workout - resistance training would involve more reps or heavier weights; circuit training would have longer work periods and/or shorter rest periods, etc.

The basic idea is to provide just enough overload/demand to create a defensive response but not too much that it overwhelms your ability to recover properly.

Summary

- ✓ **Any form of exercise should be started gradually and 'progressively' built up in both amount of 'work' and 'intensity' of effort over a period of 'time'.**
- ✓ **Too much, too quick creates the equivalent of a Sun burn rather than a Sun tan.**
- ✓ **Don't forget that sufficient recovery between workouts is vital to make progress.**
- ✓ **Age, gender, experience, goals, etc. need to be considered when determining training intensity and frequency.**

Keep pushing the limit

Unfortunately, it's not all sunshine and roses in the 'progressive overload garden' (life never is), because this particular methodology is both a boon and a curse. The good news is that it creates an ever-increasing level of improved cardio-vascular fitness, muscle tone (or mass if you're a body builder), etc. However, the bad news is that you've got to keep pushing your limits, sometimes to merely stand still, let alone make improvements.

Sadly, deep down, and despite your best intentions, your body is bone-idle and given half a chance, will revert to its previous untrained, unfit self with a proclivity for watching reruns of Jeremy Kyle and eating ice-cream, rather than undertaking energy-sapping exercise. Even if you just maintain your current training protocols (for example, you now regularly run 5k every week), then unless you find some way of stepping up your training output (increases in either frequency, time and/or intensity), something called the Law of Diminishing Returns kicks in and you start to see less results for the same effort.

Initially, you burn lots of energy (calories) whilst developing the required fitness levels to perform your weekly 5k run without collapsing in a sweat-soaked heap.

But once this level has been attained, your body will gradually learn to use less and less energy to perform the same task. So, to maintain the same energy expenditure as before, you've got to increase your training output, i.e. either run more often, run further, or run the same distance, but faster.

Tip: This can be a pretty depressing prospect: the thought of working harder and harder just to stand still, but it's not all misery and sorrow. Remember that ALL forms of exercise and activity will burn calories and fat, deplete energy stores and improve mood. More importantly, and for very important reasons we're about to explain, they stop the body from reverting into the TV watching, biscuit eating slob!

Efficient evolution

It all harks back to our early evolution. Your body is designed to be as efficient as possible and refuses to spend any more energy than is absolutely necessary. Therefore, it always, always tries to minimise cost. It's a little like a shopkeeper taking on temporary staff for the busy Christmas period and then letting them go in January when business is quiet, and he has no intention of paying anyone to just stand around doing nothing.

Likewise, the initial physiological improvements following a workout are only transient and if not repeated within the next 7-10 days, will start to 'decompensate' or regress back to their original 'untrained' state. The longer you go without working out, then the greater the regression.

However, once you've been training for a few months or years, the once-temporary changes to your heart, lungs, muscles, bones, etc. will have become more permanent and fixed into place, building the foundation for further increases to develop within the specific tissues. Basically, you won't go all the back to the beginning.

Using the shopkeeper analogy again, it would be akin to a scenario where trade has picked up after the Christmas rush and the temporary employees are still needed to cope with an increased demand. If business continues to flourish (e.g. an increase in training output) then even more staff will be required. Again, temporary at first but then making the positions permanent when the business will support it. If business drops off (e.g. a decrease in training output) then savings must be made, and staff will be sacked.

If you cease training altogether then your body eventually reverts to its pre-training levels. However, any type of exercise - regardless of its duration or intensity level – will slow down the reversing process.

Often, we've had clients who, for whatever reason, have had to cut back on their training and we simply put them on a 'maintenance' program to stop any regression. This means that when they start up again, the path to their prior fitness levels is much shorter.

This is not quite the end of the sorry 'regression' story just yet, there's one last thing. Changing your body shape, either by exercise or a dietary regime, is a steep learning-curve for your body to acclimatise to, but once it's had some practise, any subsequent attempts are easier. With exercise, this is beneficial due to a process commonly called Muscle Memory. Unfortunately, with a 'diet' a similar biological process actually works against you because your body has now learnt how to survive on fewer calories.

Note: We've very over-simplified the effects of regression on human physiology. It's highly unlikely that an athlete with five, ten or fifteen years of experience would 'regress' back to a completely untrained state. Consistent training over an extended period would cause alterations at a genetic level, which would probably never be entirely reversed, so whilst there may be some substantial regression due to a lay-off, it won't be 100 percent. This is what is commonly called, 'muscle memory': the longer a muscle has been trained for, the 'more' it remembers.

Summary
- ✓ Your body will start to gradually 'regress' from about 7-10 days after your last workout.
- ✓ Just maintaining the same training output each week has some benefits and stops regression. Ideally you should try and increase your training output when possible.
- ✓ Any type of increased activity level or specific exercise regime is better than nothing.
- ✓ The longer you've trained for, then the quicker your body returns to prior fitness levels.
- ✓ Conversely, the longer you've 'dieted', the better your body gets at living off fewer calories and therefore reducing the efficacy of further 'diets'.

Harder is not always better!

Currently, there's are very worrying trend in our industry involving Personal Trainers and other similar coaches that seem to work purely on the theory that if something is harder, then it must be better. By this logic therefore, a 1st degree burn is 'better' than a nice, healthy-looking, glowing tan.

I'll use a great example that was in the newspaper recently about some minor 'reality TV' female celebrity (are Reality-TV contestant's proper celebs?) who was doing press-ups in the mud, whilst being barked at by her boot-camp instructor (we've no idea if he was ex-forces but he was wearing army boots, so we suppose that qualifies). Fortunately, a professional photographer 'just' happened to be near-by to take some pictures*.

In what possible way can doing some press-ups in the mud produce notably better results than press-ups performed in a gym? The simple answer is that unless you are going to be in a situation that involves being good at doing press-ups in a muddy environment, they can't. This is nothing more than perpetuating the myth of the 'harder is better' route to fitness and completely ignores another vital exercise principle: Functional specificity.

Functional specificity is easily explained by demonstrating that if, for example, you want to be a good runner, don't waste too much time or effort with cycling.

In fact, this is a fundamental law of the universe. Just as two men carrying a large pane of glass must cross a road in the path of a runaway vehicle, a photographer must 'casually' walk by when a minor celebrity is training and has an exercise DVD due out. We live in a weird world don't you think!

Whilst both forms of exercise will improve both general cardiovascular capability and leg strength/fitness, the specific muscular 'function' of running is different to that of cycling. Muscles become 'fitter' by continuously and specifically performing repetitive movements under stress, so a 'fit' runner may not necessarily be a 'fit' cyclist.

Another prime example of this effect is the current obsession with core training. Core training is specifically working the muscles of the abdominal and lumbar area to improve their function. This is with the hope that the result will be an improved posture and less susceptibility to back injury, etc. This is all very good in theory but doesn't quite work as well in practice due to most core exercises being performed in a horizontal position - crunches, plank, etc. Whereas in fact, postural and back problems occur when the body is vertical, not laid flat. Therefore, the muscles are being trained to become stronger, but this improvement lends little to their actual, real life function.

This is not decrying 'core' training as useless because it isn't. but anyone that simply thinks performing 'the plank' for two minutes or doing one hundred crunches every day will solve the back, shoulder and neck problems caused by sitting in a 'slumped' position over a computer all day, is woefully mistaken.

A good example of this is what we call 'circus training': people in gyms performing weird exercises and balancing acts on fit-balls (Ann demonstrates some proper fit-ball exercises in Chapter 26).

The most ludicrous one we saw recently was a PT with a female client who was trying (and failing miserably) to perform press-ups with her feet placed on a fit-ball and her hands on a medicine ball. She couldn't even do one single press-up and when she fell off the ball for the third time the PT gave up, screaming: "Hold your core tight" at the top of his voice and promptly informed her that her 'core strength' was rubbish and needed more work! There's nothing wrong at all with trying 'balancing acts' for fun but unless you are training to be a circus performer, they have little real function in everyday life.

We've lost count of the horror stories we've heard, about individuals being so sore that they can't dress themselves the next day, not to mention the muscle tears, sprains and other injuries that are inflicted on the boot-camp and circus-training wounded.

Don't get us wrong, we've both been trained over the years by seriously tough, sadistic instructors and we're more than capable of training clients like that as well, but we are not blithely indiscriminate about who we would squeeze through that particular workout-mangle.

The upshot of this bit of waffle is that if you are making your workout tougher, ensure that it is taking a step further on your way to achieving your goals, and not just harder for the sake of it (or the fact that your personal trainer has a big mouth and wears army boots).

Okay, let's now look at the best fat-burning workouts.

*****

Chapter 27:

The best fat-burning workouts

*'Wouldn't losing weight be more fun if you could
hear the fat scream as it burned?'*
Anonymous

WE'RE GOING to let you into a little secret (but don't tell anyone else): all forms of exercise, regardless of type, duration and intensity, will burn fat! It doesn't matter if you are lifting weights, dancing or running marathons, your body will provide some of the energy you need from your fat stores. Basically, every exercise in the world could be classed as a 'fat burner'; the real – and very important - questions are:

1. Is there an optimum activity for maximising fat burning?
2. If so, how much fat is burnt off?

We mentioned earlier that our early evolution has forced humans to become highly energy-efficient, particularly with the sparing-use of our precious fat stores. The same eons-long process ensured that carbs were the main fuel used during fairly intense activity and fat sat in the background for use when intensity reduced to considerably lower levels.

To make matters worse, even at rest or very low levels of activity, humans cannot purely use fat as its only source of fuel. **At best, we only burn about 80 calories of fat per 100 calories of energy expended at rest and about 60 calories per 100 when exercising.**

With the remaining balance consisting of carbs or proteins that have been converted to carbs.

Note: your body converts all forms of carbs, from fruit to potatoes and bread to broccoli, into a simple sugar called glucose. This form of sugar is the only one that can be used for fuel. If you are not burning the glucose, it's stored in the muscles as a compound called glycogen. And if your glycogen stores are full, it is converted to fat. For simplicities sake, we'll just keep using 'carbs' as a common term.

Optimal fat-burning

So, we need to consider how best to optimise fat burning and for that we must look at how our bodies burn fat. This brings us to three more terms:

1. **Aerobic activity**
2. **Anaerobic activity**
3. **Oxygen debt**

The word aerobic means 'with oxygen' and anaerobic relates to 'without oxygen', and we'll come to oxygen debt shortly. Okay, apart from learning a little bit of pub-quiz trivia, how do these terms apply to both exercise and effective fat-burning? Using this 'with/without oxygen' classification, we can build on the information from chapter 22 (Training: the basic principles) where we discussed the intensity of a workout (walk, jog, sprint, etc.). How this is relevant to fat-burning, is to do with how hard we are breathing during training. From this we can determine which fuel is being prioritised as follows:

- ✓ **Aerobic** activity: Fat is the primary fuel during light to moderately hard breathing (where you can get most of the air that you need by breathing through your nose).
- ✓ **Anaerobic** activity: Carbs are the primary fuel when you are breathing hard to point of breathlessness and you wish you could breathe through your ears as well as your mouth,

You'll notice that we've said 'primary' fuel and not 'only' fuel. As we've just noted, this is because your cells will always use both fat and carbs for fuel. However, the important point is that as fat usage increases, sugars decrease and vice versa.

But how can you tell what you're burning at any one time?

The talk test

If you are exercising at a level of intensity that makes you breathe harder than at rest but not actually panting like a shaggy dog on a hot day, then you would be classed as training within your aerobic capacity. Therefore, fat is your primary fuel.

But if your exercise intensity rises to a point where you feel a burning sensation in the working muscles and your heartbeat is elevated high enough to feel it pounding in your ears, then you are anaerobic, and carbs are the main fuel. At these higher intensity levels your muscles are now writing cheques that your heart and lungs cannot cash. This is called oxygen debt. In other words, your muscles are now 'owed' some oxygen and this is also why you carry on breathing hard even when you've stopped exercising - your muscles are claiming the extra oxygen they are due.

The easiest way of working this out without using heart rate monitors, phone apps, etc. is to try the 'talk test'. If, whilst exercising, you can still talk without any serious pauses, you're aerobic; if not, and you can't talk and train, you're anaerobic.

Tip: If you try talking to yourself whilst out running through the local park, people may think you're a bit of a nutter, so try whistling instead. If you can't whistle in the first place, put on some headphones and hopefully any passers-by will think you're talking 'hands free'!

Oxygen debt

Sorry, but we're going to dip into a bit of science to explain about oxygen debt. However, it's worth reading because it will explain how virtually every 'fat-busting' claim made by people and companies with a vested interest in lightening your wallet, not your waistline, is utter and complete nonsense.

We touched on this earlier but it's worth mentioning again. On average, humans burn about five calories per litre of oxygen they metabolise.

Note: this is what the cells use, not what gets through your lungs because not all the oxygen may be used. As you get fitter you will metabolise a far greater percentage of the oxygen that you breathe in.

Now, firstly, our cells directly don't 'burn' oxygen in the same way that a naked flame does. Instead, we use it to recycle waste compounds from the cell as it produces energy. (This is not dissimilar to the exhaust system of a car which removes waste gases from the engine.)

The incredibly complex energy processes within the cell involves two main elements: carbon and hydrogen, both of which we get from the breakdown of sugars and fats. Once they've been used by the cell during energy metabolism, they become waste compounds. These then must be removed as soon as possible, and this is where oxygen comes in. If you mix carbon and oxygen, you create carbon di-oxide or CO_2 which we then breathe out.   Likewise, mixing oxygen with hydrogen creates H_2O or water, which is reabsorbed back into the body for further use.

As your intensity levels increase, so does the demand for energy, which in turn, draws more carbon and hydrogen (sugar and fats) into the cell. Without sufficient oxygen to remove the build-up of waste carbon and hydrogen, energy production soon stops and so do you! With aerobic activity, the intensity of effort is low enough to allow oxygen to remove the waste compounds before they cause a problem, allowing you to maintain your activity. However, at anaerobic intensities, waste products build-up faster than they can be removed.

At this point you'll feel a 'burning sensation' within the working muscles, which can become excruciating if you try to maintain the intensity.

Note: The nerdy–bit is now over but if you're interested to learn more about how your aerobic capacity is calculated, just Google something called 'VO2 max' - it will keep you entertained for hours whilst you try and decipher it. (I think it's seriously nerdy, so I haven't even tried to explain it to you!) Also, don't think you can burn more calories just by sitting in a chair and taking lots of deep breaths (you'll very likely hyper-ventilate and pass out); remember, we're talking about what you use, not just what you breathe in.

How oxygen debt relates to fat-burning is simple: carbs can burn with or without oxygen being present, but fat can't! Fat needs oxygen to be used as a fuel and when your muscles are in 'debt' to oxygen, it means there is not enough available and the amount of fat you burn drops dramatically.

Summary
- ✓ **From all this oxygen-based mumbo-jumbo, we can say that the optimum fat burning activities fall under the aerobic category - power-marching, jogging, dancing, etc.**

How much fat can you burn in a workout?

So, we've established that aerobic activity is the best option for fat burning but unfortunately, we may have been asking the wrong question. More importantly, we need to consider the second question that we posed at the beginning of this chapter: how much fat does your workout burn? And the answer is, very little.

Sadly, even the most effective 'fat-burning' routines would need to be performed for at least 8-10 continuous hours (probably more) before they accounted for the loss of just 1lb (0.5kg) from your unwanted wobbly bits.

So, Davina or whichever celebrity has a training DVD out may tell you that it's a fat-blaster of a programme but fail to mention that you'll need to do it all day to see a noticeable difference in fat reduction.

Note: at this point we'd just like to remind you that we are still talking about fat-burning, not calorie burning. If you can recall, we've already noted that the harder you breathe, then the more calories you burn. And we'll now explain how this works because we're going to discuss the fat burning zone.

Tip: we're often asked: "What's the best piece of exercise equipment to use for weight/fat loss?" The answer is very simply the one you would enjoy using the most (or certainly dislike the least). Technically, a treadmill or an exercise bike is probably the most effective at fat burning because only the legs are really working and they're the best fat burning muscles in the body. Rowing, cross (elliptical) trainers and stair climbers such as a Versaclimber, involve the use of upper body as well as lower body muscles, so they're slightly better suited for overall fitness. However, as you've just read, it's such a tiny difference to the amount of fat you actually burn, the best choice is pick the one that's less of a chore. That way, you're more likely to put in both more effort and use it more often than something you hate using.

The fat-burning zone

If you are training aerobically, then about 60% of the calories you burn will come from your fat cells, with the rest from sugars stored within the muscles and liver (plus a small amount of protein converted to sugar as well). But, as you're not breathing very hard, then overall calorie burning will be fairly low.

Once you step up the pace and you start to get out of breath, then your calorie expenditure goes up. But because there is less oxygen available to the cells, the amount of fat burnt starts to drop. At just outside your aerobic capacity (talking gets a little harder), it drops to about 50% and if the pace gets higher (talking is possible but difficult) it drops to about 40%.

And when you're training at a pace where talk is impossible, it's as low as 15%. However, this breathless intensity level is not possible to maintain for more than about a minute. So, once the pace or intensity drops, and your oxygen debt reduces (you can talk again), using fat for fuel kicks back in.

Now here's the weird thing:

Regardless of the intensity of the training, the actual amount of total fat you burn during the workout will be about the same (eh…what??).

Let's assume you're an average person with a moderate level of fitness and you hit the treadmill and jog (6mph) for an hour. You're not completely out of breath during the run, so you're within your aerobic capacity. Therefore, you're in the optimum fat burning zone, averaging about 700 calories per hour energy expenditure. At 60% fat burning this would mean you've used approx. 420 calories from your fat stores (700 x 60% equals 420).

Note: Burning 420 calories' worth of fat would mean you're now about 1.7 ounces (47g) lighter; weight-wise, this would be equivalent to a decent dollop of mayonnaise (fat has 9 calories per gram, so 420 divided by 9 equals 47g). Also, 1pound of fat has 3,500 calories of energy and at an hourly rate of 420 'fat' calories per hour, you would have to jog over 8-hours to lose, what would be just a tiny, tiny portion of your wobbly bits.

Now let's run for an hour (8-9mph), rather than jog.

You've been breathing harder throughout the hour and you're now hitting about 900 calories per hour. However, because carbs have contributed more energy, your fat burning percentage has dropped to about 45%, which means you are still burning about 400 calories of fat during the hour (900 x 45% equals 405).

You can take it a stage further and put in some 60 seconds, all-out sprints. At times, you've been breathing so hard you've almost swallowed your tongue and wish you had the ability to breathe through your ears.

You've now run off 1,200 calories and fat burning has dropped even lower to average out over the hour at about 30-35% but this still equals 360-420 calories-worth of wobbly bits (1,200 x 30/35% equals 360/420).

In all three cases, the hour on the treadmill has roughly used-up the same amount of fat but if you remember from the previous chapters, intense bouts of exercise increase your metabolic rate for a sustained period after the workout has finished. (Remember, this extra bit of metabolism may or may not amount to much - possibly 50-200 calories over the next 24-48 hours - but over time, this would add up to thousands of calories.)

Plus, with the tougher runs, you've also burnt off a lot more calories and depleted your carb stores by a greater degree. This is important when you are trying to lose weight because this means there's less chance of any carbs eaten after your workout 'over-spilling' into your fat stores. Even better, because you're pushing your heart and lungs a bit harder, your fitness levels (as well as health) improve at a faster rate. This effect is not just restricted to cardiovascular exercises such as running or cycling but it also extends to circuit training, weights, etc.

So, this has been a complicated chapter and we'll have a quick summary before we move on to working out how to perform a workout.

Summary

✓ **The fat-burning zone is a misconception.**
✓ **All activity, regardless of intensity burns fat to some degree.**
✓ **Optimum fat burning activities fall under the aerobic category - power-marching, jogging, dancing, etc**
✓ **However, high intensity activity accounts for more calories burnt during the workout.**
✓ **Whilst overall fat burning may be low during high intensity activity, it may be increased for up to 48 hours afterwards.**

****

Chapter 28:
Deciding what to do

'The hardest workout you'll ever do is getting off the couch'.
Paul & Ann

SO, WE'VE had a chat about demand, overload, recovery, modification, etc. We've discussed how long to train (volume), as well as how hard (intensity) and hopefully, you should now have a clearer picture about the metabolic effects of exercise (especially fat burning). But, how does this all fit together in a programme? Well, get those trainers out of the cupboard because in this chapter, it's time to look at what type of exercise to do.

Set your targets

So far, we've discussed quite a bit of theory about exercise - overload, work, intensity, etc. But that's just been setting the background for this chapter, which will try and explain what you should (or should not) be doing in the way of a workout.

The first thing you need to do is decide what your primary goals are.

✓ Do you just want to lose weight and burn body fat?

✓ Do you want to tone up as well?

✓ Are there specific body parts that you want to pay more attention to?

✓ Do you have a specific goal in mind such as running a half-marathon or improving your strength/stamina for a specific sport?

These are very important questions to determine from the outset, otherwise the words, 'chicken' and 'headless' become appropriate. If you have more than one goal, then write them down in order of priority.

Once you've got your list, decide how much time you have available each week to do some exercise. Most of all, be realistic. Yes, in an ideal world you may think you could do an hour a day but in the real world, it may be an hour every other day. Don't set ridiculous targets, like getting up at 5.30am every morning to run for 45 minutes if you've already got a hectic lifestyle.

Tip: set an absolute minimum weekly amount and anything else is a bonus. Use a calendar to note every session that you hope to accomplish and mark them accordingly as you either complete or miss them. At the end of the month you will have a visual record of how achievable they've been and then you can plan the next month.

You'll probably find many of your goals overlap, for instance, you may want to lose weight/fat, get fitter and run a 10k charity race. In this example, a simple running programme can achieve all three goals.

However, you may want to tone your arms (banish the bingo-wings). Possibly you want firmer Pecs (men: just say NO to moobs) shoulders and tummy as well. Sadly, running will do nothing to shape the upper body at all.

Therefore, you're going to have to put aside time for some form of resistance training to get the shape you want. At this point, let's have a look at the general types of workouts, that as an individual, you may wish to consider (we're not going to talk about team sports or anything sports specific – boxing, martial arts, etc.). Whilst there are millions of exercise forms, routines, workouts, etc. they can all be covered by two broad categories (although they can overlap).

1. Cardio-vascular (CV)
2. Resistance

Cardio-vascular training (CV)

CV training is designed to benefit and improve the working capacity of the heart and lungs. From a health point of view, it's certainly the overall king-of-the-hill workout. In the last chapter we explained that all exercise burns fat to a greater or lesser degree, but it's generally accepted that CV training covers both fat-burning as well as fitness (depending on how hard you train). In fact, in many circles, a fat-burning workout is commonly referred to as 'doing some CV'.

It's usually performed for at least 30 minutes (your body's fat burning systems don't get up to full speed for the first 10-15minutes) and up to 60 or 90 minutes with little or no rest stops to maintain an elevated heart rate. Generally, the pace is steady, with occasional bouts of higher intensity work (called intervals).

There are numerous ways of performing a CV workout: treadmill, bike, cross-trainer, stepper, spinning, aerobic, dance classes, etc. But if you don't have access to equipment then you can simply try the following options.

Power-marching

This is very likely the simplest, cheapest and most effective way of increasing your activity. You don't need any equipment other than a comfortable pair of shoes and you can pretty much do it anywhere at any time.

Power-marching is basically walking at the fastest pace that you can without breaking into a run (note: we're not talking about speed-race walking, where competitors waddle about looking like their bum is trying to chew a toffee).

When you set off, imagine that you're very late for something and you need to get a move on.

Impact wise, power-marching is much friendlier on the knees, hips and ankles than jogging or running because you always have one foot on the floor. Therefore, there's less body-weight coming down on the front foot when it lands.

This means it causes far less post-workout soreness, and it can be performed on a regular basis. It's a great activity for anyone, regardless of age, gender and current fitness level.

Jogging/Running

We regularly hear people tell us that they intend to take up jogging or running to get fit. (Note: the difference between jogging and running is simply the pace you move at. Jogging is a slower pace with a shorter stride length and running is faster, with a definite push off the front foot to increase stride length).

What they don't realise however, is that you've got to be pretty fit in the first place to start running. In fact, looking at a lot of the people around Sheffield that we see 'jogging/running' along, we feel like stopping them and telling them to walk before they have a coronary! Also, their running style is so bad, you can almost hear their knees screaming for mercy.

When you walk, there is about one and a half times your body weight on the knees and ankles but when you run, this increases to about five times your body weight. However, this all depends on your natural gait and how fast you are travelling, so it's open to question about the true amounts. Regardless, running places a strain on your lower limbs.

We're not saying don't jog or run but if you're carrying a lot of weight, have not run for ages or even hate the thought of pounding the pavements, then the benefits of jogging or running will probably not outweigh the costs to your joints and health. If, however, you feel comfortable when you run, then it's a great way to burn off some calories.

Cost-wise, apart from buying some decent quality trainers, you're on your way.

Cycling

Now we're getting into increasing the financial cost of exercise, as the first thing you need for cycling is to buy a bike and for safety's sake a helmet as well.

You may also need lights and a padlock and chain, not to mention the optional day-glow Lycra clothing.

Tip: If you're already rake-thin and super fit, it's reasonably acceptable but if you've got a few wobbly bits, you may resemble a condom trying to restrain a jelly! Trust us, it's not a good look.

The major pros for cycling are that again, it's a great way to burn calories and get fit and it's much easier on the joints. If you can cycle in the countryside, it's a lovely way to while away a few hours but when you cycle in a built-up (urban) area, you may have to consider the possibility of an unpleasant visit to the A&E Department of your local hospital.

According to the Royal Society for the Prevention of Accidents (ROSPA), in the UK in 2016 there were 18,477 reported accidents, including 102 fatalities and 3,397 serious injuries. These are only the accidents reported to the police and ROSPA estimate the total number of overall injuries to be two or three times higher.

We are not in the business of 'cyclist-bashing' and we're well aware of the improvements to the climate and air quality if everyone ditched cars in favour of bikes. But this book purely deals with the various pros and cons of exercise, not the morals and politics of the modern world at large.

Again, you must consider if the benefits outweigh the cost but a simple option (and often cheaper) is to buy an exercise bike for use indoors (then you can wear as much Lycra as you like!).

Swimming

Swimming is also a great way to burn calories and improve your fitness. Plus, it's easy on the joints as well. Obviously, you need access to a pool but don't be afraid to add some swimming into your training regime.

CV and the TOFI trainer!

Before we talk about resistance training, we just want to mention what happens if you train too much CV.

Whilst there will always be great health benefits from CV work, there's no guarantee that you will get in shape. Yet, we've very rarely ever seen anyone that doesn't respond to a resistance-based programme.

But trust us on this, we've seen many hundreds of people over the years that put in hour after hour of running, aerobics, step/dance classes, spinning, etc. and they never seem to change shape at all. It may be that they just do hours of CV work to counter balance the effects of a poor diet. But it's more likely that because CV based training will never develop any muscle tone to any noticeable degree - especially in the upper body - they just always look soft and flabby. This is what we call a thin/fat person or generally referred to as a TOFI - Thin Outside Fat Inside.

Is this you? Do you have a decent diet and spend hours on the treadmill and cross-trainer and never see any change? If it is, then you are probably not responding to CV training and you will need to try some type of resistance or circuit-type training if you want to see some results. There's no need to stop doing all your CV work, just don't do as much and try something else instead.

If you still find concept hard to grasp, let's give you one more reason: one pound of body fat contains approx. 3,500 calories of energy, whereas one pound of muscle tissue has about 700 calories (mainly because muscle tissue is about 70% water, with the remaining 30% consisting of proteins and carbs). Now, one of the easiest ways for your body to become 'better' at CV training is to become lighter - simply because you're not hauling as much weight about.

Now at first, this may sound like a clever idea, but it doesn't take a maths genius to work out that your body can lose five pounds of muscle for every pound of body fat to 'lighten up' and achieve an improved efficiency for CV work. The upper body is the prime candidate for any muscle loss because these are the muscles that are being 'carried by the legs (because they don't really contribute towards the workout, their muscle mass is not needed).

Paul Lonsdale & Ann Hirst

Now don't panic, doing a couple of hours a week on the treadmill is not going to create the problem. No, we're discussing people who do more than five or six hours of nothing but CV work per week. There's nothing wrong with training for an hour a day if you have the time - and the energy - just don't make it all CV work.

Resistance training (weights)

With resistance training, you are generally targeting specific muscles or muscle groups, thereby improving their strength, shape and tone. The most common forms of resistance training involve the use of weights, but you can also just as easy use your own body weight, e.g. press-ups or resistance bands/tubes or even household objects such as broom handles or tins of beans.

Resistance training is often very misunderstood as to its effects due to its association with heavy weights and body-building. Many people, especially women, seem concerned that they will 'bulk up' if they lift weights and this is simply not true. The primary cause of 'bulking up' is eating too much food. Body-building is at the extreme end of the resistance-training spectrum - it's like comparing a jog round the park to ultra-marathon running.

A properly designed resistance program will improve both the shape and tone of the muscles, increase bone density and tendon/ligament strength, as well as increasing your metabolic rate. If you want to look toned and tight, as opposed to soft and flabby, then some form of resistance training is an absolute must!

Why everyone should train with weights

But, why should you develop lean muscle? Well, the answer is simple: weight for weight, muscle burns about 3-4 times as much energy as fat.

Over the years, there have been numerous studies conducted which suggest that muscle burns up to thirty-times more energy than fat but most of these studies have since proven to be flawed. Current research suggests that one pound (about 0.5kg) of muscle will burn between 6-10 calories per day as opposed to an equivalent amount of fat, which is around the 2-4 calories per day mark.

The other thing to consider is that if you are overweight, then fat will not just be stored under the skin and in the abdomen, it will also run in thick veins throughout your muscle tissue as well (you can see this quite clearly on cheaper cuts of meat).

Therefore, as your fat levels reduce, so will the amount that runs through the muscle, leaving it leaner and harder but not bigger!

Note: In our hearts, we are weight trainers. We always, always introduce some type of resistance/weight training to our clients. Men generally enjoy the challenge of lifting weights, but as we've just mentioned, many women are averse to weight training. Often just suggesting to one of our female clients that she should try weight training is akin to asking her to sell one of her children! However, we persevere with their conversion and without exception, **they love it!** They love how their muscles feel after the workout. They love how their clothes fit better; they love the rapid shape-improving results they get, often after years of just doing nothing but CV-type training. Also, we think they also enjoy the feeling of belonging to an almost exclusive and secret sisterhood of like-minded women who 'weight train'!

Unlike CV training, which attempts to maintain an elevated heart rate, resistance training is performed in short, but intensive bursts called sets. Each set is taken to a point where the actual exercise is very difficult to endure any further.

The common terminology for resistance training is sets and reps; a single move is called a 'rep' and a series of continuous reps are called a set, i.e. one press-up would be a rep and ten press-ups without pause would be a set. Often, the sets are repeated 2-3 times until no further reps can be performed.

For example, you may wish to do 30 press-ups but can only manage 10-12 before your strength runs out (and even a personal trainer with a red-hot poker threatening to apply it to your soft-nether regions would not make you do any more). In this case you would break the exercise down into more manageable chunks of sets of 10 reps. At the end of each set, you would pause for a short period of 30-60 seconds and then repeat for another 10 reps, rest again and repeat until you achieved your target of 30 reps.

Circuit or interval training

We've listed circuit/interval training in its own category because it can be both CV and resistance based. Generally, the exercises are performed against a stop-watch, as opposed to sets and reps and each exercise is called a 'station'. A circuit would be comprised of anything between 5-20 stations of various exercises.

For example:

Station 1: Press-ups

Station 2: Lunges

Station 3: Abdominal crunches

Station 4: Star Jumps

Station 5: Bench dips

Station 6: Shuttle runs

The exercise at each station would be performed for a pre-determined time-period - anything between 20-60 seconds - followed by a very short rest (10-30 seconds) and then on to the next station. Once an entire 'circuit' of stations had been completed, there would be a longer rest period and either the same circuit repeated or a new one set up.

The best circuit-routines involve a series of stations that alternate between muscle groups to allow for a minimum rest period, i.e. in the above circuit, press-ups (upper-body) are followed by lunges (lower-body), followed by abs (core), etc. The objective is to get as many reps out at each station for as long as you can until either the time is up, or your muscles can no longer carry on.

Therefore, it falls under both CV and resistance - the heart-rate is continuously high due to the volume of work and little rest-time, but the muscles are failing from the intensity of the particular exercise.

For someone trying to lose weight, get fit, burn calories and develop muscle tone, circuit or interval training is ideal.

High Intensity Interval Training (HIIT)

At this point we'd just like to mention the latest fitness trend doing rounds, something called 'HIIT'. You may or may not have heard of this, but regardless, it's a very effective method of improving fitness, stamina and increasing post-workout metabolism. However, it is being slightly over-sold, with claims of just three minutes every other day as the cure-all for all weight (and health) problems. However, HIIT is not a new idea. In fact, ask any body builder or boxer of any experience and they'll say: "Been there, done that!"

The idea is to train at a maximum pace for a short period of time – 20-30 seconds – followed by a similar rest period and then repeat for as many rounds as possible. Note: when we say maximum, we mean full-on, spleen-busting, all-out effort. Imagine the, 'you're being chased by a bear' type of effort and intensity.

We have our own version called 20/20 training.

20/20 training

You can do this type of workout with any exercise you wish. You could sprint, use a piece of cardio equipment, or simply use resistance tubes, dumb bells or a multi-gym.

Each round comprises 20 seconds of effort with a 20 second rest period. Immediately following this rest period, you start the next round. Basically, it's continuous 20 seconds on/off until you've completed anywhere from five to eight rounds (depending upon current fitness levels). The whole workout takes between three and five minutes to complete.

We have three ways of doing this:

Straight sets for five-eight rounds

✓ Pick a weight or tension on a resistance tube (or level on a bike, cross trainer, etc.) and try to maintain both number and speed of reps for all rounds. Do not change the weight/tension throughout and if you get it right, the first two or three rounds will not be too hard but the final few rounds are killers.

Descending sets for five-eight rounds

✓ The aim is to keep the same number of reps at each round, working at maximum from round one. Start at the heaviest weight/tension you can manage for twenty seconds and reduce gradually at each round to maintain rep output.

Pyramid sets for ten rounds

✓ Start with less weight/tension and increase by small increments until you max out at round five or six. Then reverse the process, gradually reducing the weight/tension over the final four or five rounds.

It helps if you can see a clock or you have a stopwatch but if not, you could just perform a set number of reps (at least ten) for each round and then take ten deep breaths for your rest period. If you want to make it harder, just amend the number of rounds or add more time to the working period or take time off the rest period.

We mix 20/20 routines with other types of training for about an hour.

For example, we'll start with a cardio 20/20 set, then possibly some upper body weights (3-4 sets of 10-12 reps), then back to a 20/20 on abs, then weights, then 20/20, and so on until the session is over. This incorporates absolutely everything into one workout.

Note: By the time you're reading this, it's highly likely that something else will have become the 'workout flavour of the month' - possibly running backwards! Actually, we're not kidding; this is termed 'retro-running' or 'retro-locomotion' and apparently is gaining popularity in some London parks. We can't wait to see the 'You've been framed' clips of that one going wrong!

Suspension training

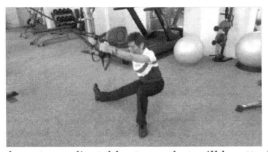

Unless you are already a member of a gym, it's unlikely you'll have heard much about suspension training.

Basically, you can perform an almost infinite amount of body weight exercises by hanging from two adjustable straps that will be attached to an anchor point on a wall, door or suitable post. All the major muscle groups (and some of the minor ones as well) can be targeted with phenomenal precision and the best part is that it always hits the core muscles regardless of whatever body part you're training.

Without doubt, it's one of the best pieces of all-body training equipment we've ever come across, but it has one slight drawback: it needs proper tuition to get it right. We've had dozens of clients who've tried it in a gym but can't seem to get the workout right (it doesn't help that some brands are fiddly to adjust for height, etc.).

However, once they've been shown how to hold the core properly and keep the hands or feet in the right line, they absolutely love the workout.

We teach a massive amount of suspension training but we're not going to show any suspension exercises in this book because you really must experience it to appreciate just how it works. However, we have a great video on our website that you can have a look at if you want to consider it for yourself.

Okay, what doesn't work?

On the flip-side from something that works well to one that doesn't, brings us to the Vibro or Power Plate. Again, if you've not heard of this it's basically a vibrating platform that you stand on a variety of positions and perform some exercises, such as press ups or squats. The idea is that because of the vibration, the exercise is much harder to perform (remember, however, that harder is not necessarily better). Now, it's not that there isn't some benefit from using a power-plate, it's just the ridiculous claims that they make. Such as: 'Just 10 minutes on our power-plate is equal to an hour in the gym' (this may well be true if you usually spend most of your time in the juice-bar watching TV!).

A reasonably tough, productive hour of mixed gym work (resistance & CV) will burn anywhere between 600-1,000 calories of energy (an average of 10-16 calories per minute) depending upon intensity, age, gender, bodyweight, etc.

So, following the Power Plate's claim to its logical conclusion, you should be able to burn an equal amount of energy in just ten minutes – an average energy expenditure of 60-100 calories per minute. Trust us, if you could burn energy at this rate, you would become so hot, your clothes would catch fire and your head will probably explode. Yet we've rarely seen anyone who uses one even break into a sweat!

To put this silly claim into perspective, running at a speed of just over 12mph (19kph) – basically an all-out sprint to a normal person - would only burn energy at about 20 calories per minute. We think someone's been rather economical with the truth!

Finally, we're going to have a quick chat about the type of person you are.

Recreational or professional athlete?

When we first interview a new, potential client, we'll initially ask about aims, goals, etc., but then we ask two more:

1. Are you doing this to make yourself feel better?
2. Are you doing this to compete in an event or at a high level in sport?

There is a very specific reason for determining where your answers fall within those questions. If your reason is purely question 1, then your workouts should be challenging and moderately difficult.

Therefore, unless you are a pain-driven, humiliation-seeking sadomasochist, they should never become a near-death experience! You're trying to feel better about life, so how can training to the point of utter exhaustion, vomiting, going temporarily blind or not being able to move for a week improve your life – it doesn't!

However, if your reasons fall within question 2, then the approach to your workouts take on a different aspect. If you wish to 'compete' at something, even if you're only competing with yourself (improving your time in a 10k for example), then you need to develop a type of mental toughness as well as physical strength, stamina, etc. to ensure you are pushing your boundaries as far as possible.

Obviously, your reasons may fall within both questions, because some people are naturally competitive, and the pleasure/pain/reward circuitry of your brain may need some amount of self-punishment to feel better. Regardless, don't lose sight of why you started and remember one of our earlier quotes:

'All exercise comes at a cost but that doesn't mean it also comes with a benefit'.

Okay, we've checked out what to do, let's have a look at where to do it.

*****

Chapter 29:
Deciding where to do it

'Losing weight means you'll look good in clothes. Training means you'll look good naked!'
Paul & Ann

UNLESS YOU ARE a totally dedicated athlete, or you already have an undying love of physical activity, undertaking any form of exercise for most people requires a serious amount of will power. It's always easier to find more reasons not to train than to get yourself going: it's raining; I'm tired; the dog needs feeding; I really need to organise the plasters (Band-Aids) in the first aid box into correct size order, etc., etc.

Therefore, it's important to find the type of training you enjoy most because you're more likely to keep up the workouts. Yet, there's another factor to consider as well: the place where you train. Again, we're not going to discuss team events or sports specific activities, which are likely to have their own specific venues, but we'll have a look at the options and pros and cons of either training in a public gym or at home.

Joining a gym

So long as you can be bothered to go, joining a gym can be very cost-effective (we've already mentioned that over £45million is wasted on gym memberships in the UK).

Obviously, it depends on overall costs but there is a new trend towards budget-priced gyms in the UK, with fees for less than £20 per month, but apart from price, there are two other major considerations:

1. Facilities and equipment
2. Locality

Earlier we mentioned that it's important to determine your primary goals and this is vital in selecting the right type of gym. There's little point in going to a 'spit and sawdust' body-building gym, full of weights and reeking of sweat-fuelled testosterone, which has one bike and an old treadmill if your aim is to perform mainly CV work and tone up your arms. Likewise, a 'fancy-pants' facility, full of Lycra and headbands and smelling like the perfume department of Harrods, may have hundreds of treadmills, bikes, etc. But if it only has one bench with 5kg dumbbells, it's useless if you want to put on some muscle.

There will be other considerations as well, such as:

✓ Opening hours
✓ Swimming pool
✓ Fitness classes: Body pump, spinning, circuits, boxercise, etc.
✓ Crèche facility

Gyms of any type can be extremely intimidating to someone with little or no training experience, so it's important, not only to find the right facilities, but a friendly atmosphere as well. You wouldn't buy expensive clothes or shoes without trying them on first, so insist on a few trial sessions and 'try before you buy' to make sure you feel comfortable with the place.

Note: In the UK, many gym contracts are, in fact, credit agreements. As such, they can be enforced under the Consumer Credit Acts if you try to cancel, so check the small print for cancellation rights. The UK government has promised to investigate the unfair practises of these types of contracts, but it may be some time before any legislation is passed.

Locality is also important. Although the gym you like may have every facility you need, if it's miles across town, the thought of the trek will be the metaphorical final nail in the reasons not to train coffin.

All things being equal, always, always pick the gym that's the most convenient to get to, especially if you are going either before or after work.

Picking a good personal trainer

Sadly, we're going to cover one last point about joining a gym: using a personal trainer. Now it goes without saying that we're a little biased about this topic. When we first started our careers in the gym, there was no such thing as a personal trainer; there was either a gym instructor or a class teacher (aerobics, step, etc.).

The main duty of the gym instructor was to be on the gym floor, ensuring everyone was training safely and effectively. He/she was there for help, advice and motivation as well as designing programmes for members **free of charge** (this service was always included in the membership).

When I first passed my City and Guilds in sport and exercise in 1983 (a 12-month part-time course) I wasn't even allowed to design programmes.

Even though I'd been weight training for over three years, I could only teach inductions to new members.

I spent most of my time studying, as well as hanging on to every word uttered by both the senior instructors and many of the incredibly fit and muscular members that acted as my mentors. About 12 months later, I was finally allowed to do basic programme design, eventually working my up to a senior position over the next few years.

Ann's story is not dissimilar and the point we are trying to make is not an 'old codger's moan about the 'young-un's' today (e.g. Monty Python's four Yorkshiremen sketch - if you can remember that far back).

However, it is now possible to go from never stepping foot in a gym to becoming a fully qualified personal trainer in about six weeks! In fact, you can now become a personal trainer via numerous online courses and the only time you walk in the gym is when you take your exams.

Don't get us wrong, there will be some very experienced and passionate personal trainers out there, but they will be far outnumbered by those who wouldn't even have the wherewithal to serve burgers and a coke, let alone design complex, tailored workouts. If and when you decide to use a personal trainer at a gym, then please consider the following questions first:

1. Do they have experience in designing the type of programme for your training goals?
2. Are they, or have they ever been in shape themselves? Training is not a theory session. To teach it properly, you must be able to do it yourself.

If the answer is no to either of the above, then look for someone else (or negotiate a really good price!).

Training at home

The idea of being able to do a workout without leaving your house is often appealing. Sadly, in our experience the drop-off rate of starting a home-based programme and then quitting within weeks is remarkably high. We used to sell home use gym equipment, so we have a lot of experience in the home training market and we don't think we'd be exaggerating if we said that 95 out of every 100 pieces sold will end up simply gathering dust in the house or being used as an ad hoc clothes horse!

This ranges from treadmills and multi-gyms right through to the ridiculous 'get a six pack in six weeks abs trimmers' that are sold in the millions on the shopping channels, as well as the worthless celebrity fitness DVD's that come out in time for Christmas.

Tip: Don't ever buy a weight loss book/DVD as a gift for a loved one. The recipient will automatically assume that you're suggesting they're fat! Even if they keep going on about losing weight, it doesn't mean that they are asking you to agree with them. It's as bad as answering yes to the question, 'does my bum look big in this?'

Regardless of all this however, if you decide to train at home you'll be surprised by how little equipment you need for a fitness/toning style workout in the front room or garage. We often train clients in their own house and all we take are:

- ✓ Resistance tubes
- ✓ Swiss or fit-ball
- ✓ A set of dumb bells up to 10kg
- ✓ An exercise mat

Resistance tubes

Tubes (or bands) are simple, but highly versatile and effective training aids. We prefer the tubes to bands because they have handles, which make them easier to use, but the principle is the same: the more you stretch them, the more tension you must overcome. They are very safe and easy to use (unless you don't anchor them properly and they 'twang' you). Plus, they are light and small enough to carry around in a small bag or hand luggage, so you can use them anywhere.

They generally come in a variety of 3-4 colours, each indicating a different strength (some manufacturers will vary in the colour/strength range) but don't underestimate them just because they're basically a big rubber band. Price-wise, they're extremely low cost and you can buy them individually or in complete sets (Amazon do a full set for about £25 or singles from about £7).

They're ideal for fitness and toning workouts, especially circuit training. But many of our body-building clients will use them to add tension to specific exercises.

The look on their faces and the subsequent groans are very satisfying, especially when Ann chides them by saying, "What's up, it's only a bit of elastic".

You can train every muscle in the body and whatever exercise you can perform with dumbbells, you can copy with tubes. As we mentioned, the greater the stretch, the greater the tension, so all you need to do is either move your foot position or step further away from the anchor point to make the workout more challenging.

All you need to do is wrap the tube around a suitable sturdy fixture or you can use a clever little accessory called a door anchor (available separately or included if you buy a complete set), which allows you safely fasten the tube to the door.

On the next page, Ann demonstrates just a few of the basic moves

Chest & back workout

✓ Perform 3-4 sets of 10-15reps with 30 seconds rest

✓ Chest: step forward to increase tension as required

✓ Back: step backwards to increase tension

Exercise	Start	Finish	Target Muscles
Chest Press			Chest, shoulders & triceps
Chest Fly's			Chest & shoulders
Double arm row			Arms & back
Single arm row			Arms & back
Pull down			Back & triceps

Shoulders & arms workout

✓ Perform 3-4 sets of 10-15reps with 30 seconds rest
✓ Front raise: take feet wider to increase tension
✓ Shoulder press: use two feet and take wider to increase tension
✓ Biceps: take feet wider to increase tension
✓ Triceps: step backwards to increase tension

Exercise	Start	Finish	Target muscles
Front raise			Shoulders
Shoulder press			Shoulders & triceps
Biceps curl			Biceps (front of upper arm)
Triceps press-down			Triceps (back of upper arm)

Lower body: glutes (bum)

- ✓ Perform 3-4 sets of 10-15reps with 30 seconds rest in between
- ✓ Side hip lift: keep knee at same angle and lift from hip
- ✓ Glutes lift: keep rear leg straight and squeeze glutes at end of lift

Exercise	Start	Finish	Target muscles
Side hip lift			Glutes & hips (bum & saddlebags)
Glutes lift			Glutes & hamstrings (rear of upper leg)

Fit balls (aka swiss balls)

Fit balls are basically a space-hopper without the handles. Although they can be used for a variety of exercises, we use mainly them for training the abs and core (see next page). Sitting (or lying) on a large inflatable ball that rolls around makes your abdominal muscles work extra hard to stabilise any wobble, ensuring a much deeper, more intense workout.

Abdominals

✓ Perform 3-4 sets of 10-15reps with 30 seconds rest

Exercise	Start	Finish	Target muscles
Abdominal crunch			Stomach - upper front area
Abdominal crunch with twist			Stomach - transverse (the bit just above the hips)
Side dip			Stomach - upper & Obliques (love-handles)
Abdominal crossover			Stomach - all areas

Core

✓ Abdominal plank: hold the position for 2-3 sets of 30-45 seconds
✓ Hip Bridge: can be performed as sets of 10-15 reps or just hold as per plank.
✓ Spread arms on floor for stability. Push hips up at same time as squeezing the glutes & abs.

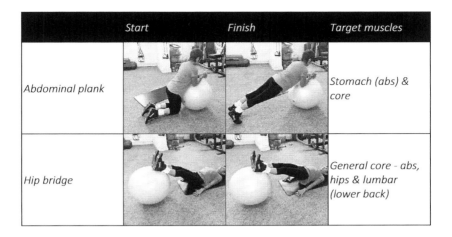

	Start	Finish	Target muscles
Abdominal plank			Stomach (abs) & core
Hip bridge			General core - abs, hips & lumbar (lower back)

These are just a few of the hundreds of options you have for training at home or in a gym. Obviously, there's no reason why you can't enjoy the best of all worlds. You can go for a jog or power-march around the local park, cycle in the countryside, use the resistance bands/fit balls at home. Then, go to a gym for classes or to use equipment that you don't have access to anywhere else.

Tip: Giving yourself as many options as possible keeps everything fresh and stops you from getting bored from doing the same activities day in day out. Don't ever be afraid to try something new - you never know; you might just enjoy it!

*****

Chapter 30:
Basic programme design

'No matter how hard you exercise, you can't train your
way out of a bad diet'
Anonymous

TO HELP MAXIMISE the time and effort you spend on your workouts, we've designed a basic template for you to follow. It's not going to cover any particular type of workout but it's the general principles of how we would put a routine together that would last between 45-90 minutes or so.

The general guide to any type of training is to:

1. **Warm up**
2. **Mobilise/loosen the muscles**
3. **Train at high intensity in the first half of the workout**
4. **Train at moderate intensity in the second half**
5. **Add a fat burning intensity level toward the end**
6. **Finish with a cool down/ abs/stretch**

Let's look at the above in slightly more detail.

1 - Warm-Up (cardio): 5minutes

✓ You only need about five minutes for the initial warm-up stage. This is to get the blood flowing and heart rate up. The first three minutes should be a steady pace, and then try to pick up the speed for the final two minutes. Ideally, you should finish the warm-up breathing relatively hard but not breathless.

✓ The best equipment to warm-up on is one that gets as many muscles as possible muscles working, e.g. rower, cross trainer, Versaclimber, etc. If you don't have any equipment, then a combination of star jumps, wall press-ups, running-on-the-spot or skipping will do just as well.

✓ At this point, you should be mentally focusing on the workout ahead - thinking about what to do and how you will do it.

✓ Unless you have a specific joint or muscle issue, spending twenty minutes on a warm-up is just wasting valuable training time.

2 - Mobility stretching (still warming- up): 5 minutes

✓ After the first warm-up, you're now going to loosen off the muscles that you are about to train. If you are doing a routine that involves every muscle group, then mobilise every muscle. If not, put greater emphasis on the muscles you are about to use.

✓ A mobility stretch only takes the muscles and joints through their normal range of movement (ROM) until you feel a moderate amount of tension – basically, it's a light stretch.

✓ At the end of the workout, you will perform some developmental stretches, where you will stretch the joint/muscle to its limit but trying to do that before you are fully warmed up is actually counter-productive.

3 - High intensity training: 15-25 minutes

✓ The idea is to perform the most arduous and taxing part of the workout in the first 25 minutes when you are strongest and freshest.

✓ This could be fitness drills, sprints on the treadmill, circuits or weights involving the major muscle groups of the legs, chest, back and shoulders.

✓ If weight training, you would use free-weights - dumb bells, barbells, etc. - at this stage.

4 - Moderate intensity training: 10-20minutes

✓ You will take the intensity down a step.

✓ At this point, your blood-sugar levels are starting to fall dramatically, and you will start to tire.

✓ Your co-ordination will worsen, increasing your chance of injury, so this is the last stage where you will do any form of exercise that requires extreme stability or balance, i.e. walking lunges, balance boards, BOSU (both sides up) balls, etc.

✓ The emphasis at this stage is moving towards smaller muscle groups, such as the arms or the use of machines instead of free-weights where you don't need to worry too much about stability.

5 - CV/Fat burning 15-30mins

✓ Depending upon your goals and available time, this is the stage where you would do a CV/fat burning routine. Your ability to use fat for fuel is minimal in the first 15 minutes of any type of workout, so it makes sense to put it towards the end, rather than the beginning of a programme.

✓ Best options are power-marching, light-jogging or cycling.

✓ Also, as your blood-sugar levels are low, your body will look towards its fat stores to make up the majority of the fuel where possible. If you are still training intensely, the conversion of proteins to carbs (sugar) will increase and you end up burning muscle off, rather than fat.

✓ In any one workout, this effect is pretty minimal and hardly noticeable but over an extended period of time, it will add up. (Remember, 1lb of fat has 3,500 calories but 1lb of muscle only has about 700 calories.)

✓ If you intend to maintain a high intensity of training beyond 45 minutes, then make sure there are some carbs still entering the bloodstream when you first start. This could be from a banana or a small bowl of cereal or toast eaten about 60 minutes before the workout (you don't want anything heavy or it may make you feel nauseous).

✓ Sports drinks such as Lucozade or Gatorade will also maintain sugar levels but if you intend to burn fat at this point, consuming a sugary drink will not help - stick to water if possible.

✓ You could also use this stage for a cool-down as well.

6 - Abdominal work/ Developmental stretching: 5-10 minutes

✓ We generally fit abs into the end of a workout but it's a personal preference option as you can fit them in wherever you wish.

✓ This is where you would perform a full stretch, pushing the muscles/joints to their maximal ROM.

✓ It's very important to stretch-off at the end of a workout for mental as well as physical reasons. The muscles and joints can be quite tight at this point and a good stretch will make them (and you) feel more relaxed.

✓ Whilst it's very difficult to actually increase the natural length of the muscles to any great degree, you can take the opportunity to both pull the muscle back to its usual length and also develop the ROM of the joints, which in turn allows the muscle to move much easier.

✓ For example, many people can't easily touch their toes because they think they have short hamstrings, whereas in fact, they've usually got normal length hamstrings - it's the mobility of the hip joint/pelvis/lumbar area (near where the hamstring attaches) that stops the hamstrings achieving their full length. Simple exercises to loosen the hips, etc. often results in clients being able to touch their toes for the first time in years.

✓ Incidentally, stretching should only be taken to a point of mild discomfort, not agony.

✓ It's worth noting however, that stretching doesn't reduce (to any great degree), the amount of soreness you may feel over the next few days. Delayed Onset of Muscle Soreness (DOMS) is related to something else entirely and we'll cover that now.

(Note: We've added this next section because we are often asked about muscle soreness, but please feel free to skip this part if it's not relevant)

Post workout soreness

It's usual to feel some soreness or tightness in the muscles for a few days after your workout. Quite simply, the ache is due to the muscles, tendons and ligaments adapting to the type of training you've just performed. It's referred to as DOMS[13] (Delayed Onset Muscle Soreness) and whilst the exact mechanism is not clear, the one thing it's definitely not, is lactic acid (more on that later).

When we ask a muscle to work hard we put it under stress and this causes micro tears in the muscle fibres and their surrounding tissues. The greatest damage occurs when you first perform a new move or move to a higher intensity of training, i.e. adding sprints to your jog or moving up to using heavier weights.

This is thought to be because of the increased load on the muscle during what is called its Eccentric or braking phase.

This is basically when the muscle has contracted (tightened) and is returning to its original position (relaxed) but you're still applying tension to control the move.

For example, the downward part of a biceps curl is the eccentric phase because when you lower the weight under control, the biceps are still working to create resistance; otherwise you'd just drop the weight on the floor.

Once the muscle has got used to this eccentric phase, the soreness is not so great, which is why the first couple of workouts of a new routine or programme are the most painful. Eventually, the muscle adapts to the workout and becomes less 'stressed' with subsequently little or no DOMS at all.

What is lactic acid?

Lactic Acid is produced when our cells and tissues start to convert glucose (sugar) to a usable energy source. Lactic acid is vital for energy and without it you wouldn't be able to stand up, let alone train. The production of lactic acid also stimulates the release of positive hormones such as Growth Hormone, which increases your post-workout metabolic rate. Lactic acid is also used directly by other organs such as the heart and is recycled back into glucose by the liver. So, contrary to popular myth, it is not a waste product.

What causes the soreness?

The soreness usually sets in about 12 – 24hours after the workout and disappears within a couple of days. The exact reason for this is still under serious scientific debate but it is thought to be because of either one or possibly both of the following:

1. The localised damage to the tissue causes inflammation (oedema) which then activates the pain sensors in the tissue. The swelling peaks after 24-48 hours, therefore causing the greatest pain.
2. The pain should be felt immediately but the post-workout endorphin-release (happy chemicals that are more powerful than morphine) blocks the pain signals for the first few hours after the exercise.

How do you get rid of it?

Regardless of reason for the DOMS, there's little you can do about it other than ease the pain. The tissue must repair itself and despite many alleged 'wonder-product' remedies, your body will repair itself in its own good time. Pre-workout mobilisation (not over stretching) and post-workout stretches of the muscles and joints will help but you can still get DOMS even if you stretch properly. However, you can alleviate the pain by increasing blood flow to the tissue, reducing inflammation and helping to remove any waste products. The best ways are:

1. Massage the affected area. As well as increasing local blood flow, the brain 'prioritises' signals from the sensors under the skin that detect heat and pressure before anything else, therefore blocking the deeper muscle pain receptors. This 'hides' the pain and offers mental comfort as well. A warm bath has a similar, temporary effect.

2. Perform very light movements or stretches that mimic the original exercise, again increasing blood flow to the area.

3. It is not recommended to take any type of anti-inflammatory at this point because the process that causes the inflammation also starts the repair procedure. If the pain continues past seven days however, then it may be worthwhile asking professional help, e.g. a medical practitioner or a physiotherapist about the problem.

Can it be avoided?

Not really, but it can be seriously reduced by NOT overdoing things for the first few workouts. Anyone new to training, or even experienced trainers starting on a new programme, should ease themselves gradually into it. This doesn't mean you won't feel anything at all, but any soreness will be light and not debilitating.

Being too sore after a workout is not only unnecessary but it's also counterproductive because you are unable to train maximally until the pain goes away. Sadly, excessive (and unnecessary) DOMS is often caused by inexperienced personal trainers, gym instructors and other fitness coaches with inflated egos, who seem to think that they are doing their client a disservice if they are not 'knackered' after every workout. As we've already said, exercise should not be a near death experience - it's simply a means to an end. It should improve fitness, make you faster, stronger, help you lose weight, etc. Ultimately, it should make you feel better about yourself, not worse.

Assessing progress in your workout should not be rated by how sore you feel but by how much improvement you've made. If a client is determined to feel sore after training, we offer to punch them on the nose as they leave the gym!

This is the general idea behind programme design. It's by no means the only system we use, as each programme should be tailored to an individual's goals (and abilities) but it should at least provide a place to start from.

*****

Chapter 31:
Paralysis by analysis

'It does not matter how slowly you go, as long as you do not stop'
Confucius

Strangely enough, we thought that out of all our written works, this one, Train Smarter, Not Harder would be the easiest to write due to our years of experience. Yet it turned out to be the hardest.

We fell victim to a syndrome that affects many people in all walks of life (but is especially prevalent for individuals who 'read' a lot about exercise). This is called paralysis by analysis. Basically, it's been faced with so many options and choices that it becomes almost impossible to decide what to do. This part of the book is about 20,000 words long. Yet we could easily have made it 40,000 words, possibly 50,000 if we cobbled together everything we've ever written about exercise.

So, we decided to keep to the basics and put everything else on our website where you can cherry-pick the relevant information. In addition to lots more articles about training, we've added a lot of instructional training videos that we hope you may find useful. If you'd like to know more, our contact details can be found at the end of the book.

So, before we finish with a summary of everything that you've read, let's just offer this last piece of advice.

Training-wise, you have four, simple four options:

1. **Do this**

2. **Do that**
3. **Do the other**
4. **Do nothing**

Okay, we lied. In fact, you only have three, because doing nothing is not an option if you want to be healthy and get in shape. Yes, try wherever possible to train smarter, but whatever else you do, just make sure that you train.

A few points to remember

- ✓ Whilst all exercise comes at a cost, it doesn't automatically mean it comes with a benefit.
- ✓ Just because something is harder, it doesn't always follow that it's 'better'.
- ✓ You must first apply some form of 'Demand' (physical stress) to your muscles, heart, lungs, etc. which is then followed by a period of 'Recovery' (rest, food and sleep) and finally you arrive at your destination: 'Modification (improved fitness, tone, strength, health, etc.).
- ✓ You can train long, or you can train hard, but you can't train long and hard.
- ✓ The harder you breathe the more calories you burn.
- ✓ Exercise that makes you breathless may elevate your metabolism for up to 48 hours afterwards.
- ✓ Whilst this may only be a few hundred calories at most, it will build up to a substantial amount over the forthcoming weeks and months.
- ✓ All programmes should contain a variety of exercises (work), as well as how long you do them for (time) and how much effort you put into them (intensity).
- ✓ Age, gender, experience, goals, etc. must be considered when determining effective training intensity and frequency levels.
- ✓ Any form of exercise should be started gradually and 'progressively' built up in both amount of 'work' and 'intensity' of effort over a period of 'time'.
- ✓ If not, you end up with a metaphorical Sun burn rather than a Sun tan.

- ✓ Your body will start to gradually 'regress' from about 7-10 days after your last workout.
- ✓ However, just maintaining the same training output each week has some benefits and stops regression.
- ✓ Ideally you should try and increase your training output when possible.
- ✓ The fat-burning zone is a misconception.
- ✓ All activity, regardless of intensity burns fat to some degree.
- ✓ Aerobic activity: light to moderately hard breathing (can still talk) - fat is the primary fuel.
- ✓ Anaerobic activity: breathing hard to the point of breathlessness (can hardly talk) - sugar (carbs) is the primary fuel.
- ✓ General programme design:

  a) Warm up

  b) Train at high intensity in the first half of the workout

  c) Train at moderate intensity in the second half

  d) Add a fat burning intensity level toward the end

  e) Finish with a cool down/ abs/stretch

- ✓ Don't over-analyse your workout too much.
- ✓ If in doubt remember KISS (Keep it Simple Stupid).
- ✓ Do this, do that or do the other. But don't do nothing.
- ✓ Try to find something that you enjoy. You'll do it more often and with more energy.

Right, enough about training, it's time to move on to the final chapter and set you off on the road to success.

*****

Chapter 32:
On the road to success

'If the ladder is not leaning against the right wall, every step we take just gets us to the wrong place faster'
Stephen R Cove

A FEW YEARS ago, we were sitting in a pub, having a dink and an interesting discussion with a friend about diets (yes, we do like alcohol and no, we're not perfect).

Like most people we meet he held some very common, but misconceived ideas about weight loss. So, for about an hour he suggested a range of popular 'diet' scenarios: Atkins, Dukan, Weight Watchers, low-fat, fasting, etc: And with every offering he thought he'd finally solved the problem to everyone's weight issues. Yet, we countered his proposals with why the plan would work for some individuals but not for others. At times, I suggested the pros of each diet and Ann the cons, then we'd swap over …. and then back again.

Finally, bewildered and dejected, he gave up, more confused now than when he started. "You know", he sighed, "you should write a book about this and call it, 'Want to lose weight? Just take your best guess". So, we did! (but we didn't think, 'just take you best guess' was much of title!)

But is this the case? Is dieting just guesswork?

Well, paradoxically, as hopefully you've now begun to gather, some of it is, but with an understanding of the right set of rules, most of it needn't be.

Yet, you must start somewhere, and hopefully after digesting all the information you've read in this book, you should now be able to take as much guesswork out as possible and now start down the final road to achieving your weight-loss objectives.

We hope that you're not too disappointed that this book is lacking in specifics: calorie calculations, recipes, only eat this, for breakfast, don't eat that, etc. Sorry, but we've learnt over the years that this doesn't work. It's not wrong to hope for someone to simply tell you what to do but this won't solve the problem, it just passes it to someone else to do it for you. It's the dietary equivalent of an unasked-for gift voucher (because nothing suggests that 'I can't really be bothered' better that a gift voucher!).

This is the main reason we don't simply tell anyone 'what to do'; instead we try to show them how to do it for themselves. Why? Because over the course of your lifetime, you will make tens of thousands of food choices. And if you can only eat 'this or that', how will you ever know if you can eat the other? How will you know if the latest food ideas and training routines have value or are merely another fad? Sadly, the answer is that you won't, and the weight-loss-merry-go-round will keep on turning.

You are about to take the first step on a journey that will last a lifetime. Along the way, there will be detours and dead-end streets and seemingly endless rainy days where your weight-loss targets seem to be stuck in a metaphorical traffic jam.

Nevertheless, there will also be super-fast highways and sun-filled glorious scenery where progress speeds along nicely.

With time, consistency, effort and willpower, you should reach your targets. Unfortunately, however, as we've constantly noted, the battle won't end there, it will keep going until your last breath.

But console yourself with the thought that the tricks and new habits that you discover along the way will be your ally for the inevitable times – post-holidays, Christmas, etc. – when your weight fluctuates, and you need to drop the couple of pounds that have crept back on. This is how your life will be, so you've got to learn to live with it. It happens to everyone one else (including us).

We now live according to a pattern of training and watching what we eat during the week and then we take the weekend off. We have a set of clothes that we use as markers and when they become uncomfortable, we tighten up our diets, e.g., dropping out starchy carbs and step up the power-marching during the week until they fit better.

It's all about balance and quality of life. We've finally found ours; hopefully, this book will help you to find yours.

*****

About the authors

We are neither Doctors nor Professors but life-affiliates of the school of common sense. Membership only has one rule - KISS – Keep It Simple Stupid'
Paul & Ann

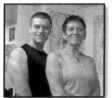 WE'VE SPENT pretty much our entire lives in the health and fitness industry. In 2002, we decided we'd had enough of working for others and set up Get Physical Ltd - our own personal training facility in Sheffield.

Despite having already busy lives, we also run an online training and dietary service, regularly lecture in and around South Yorkshire and often talk on local BBC radio.

We would love to say that in our spare time we do something exciting like paragliding, Himalayan trekking or raising money for endangered tree frogs in Patagonia. Sadly, this is not the case.

In truth, we divide our precious downtime with our families - especially our grandchildren (I've got four, Ann has two). We work in the garden (well, Ann does - the only 'garden' I enjoy is preceded by the word, 'beer').

We read, do crosswords and occasionally rant about the new-idiot-on-the-block who turns up in the media with some half-baked idea purporting to reinvent the weight-loss wheel or revolutionise the health industry (not surprisingly, this takes up much of our time).

If you were ever to meet us, you would quickly realise that health, exercise and nutrition isn't just something that we do, it's what we are.

Paul & Ann

Incidentally, most of the 'quotes' you've read throughout the book are ours (we've accredited the ones that aren't). They're bits and pieces of humour and observations that we've made over the years. We hope you've enjoyed them.

Get in touch

If you've enjoyed this book, then please feel free to post a review on Amazon or a like on your preferred social media channel: Facebook, Instagram, etc.

And if you would like any further help at all, our contact details are below:

Get Physical Ltd

Millennium House

30 Junction Road

Sheffield, S11 8XB

Tel: 0114 2666433

Web: www.winningtheinchwar.com

Email: info@winningtheinchwar.com

*****

Index

References

[1] *https://nutritionandmetabolism.biomedcentral.com/articles/10.1186/s12986-018-0249-z*

[2] www.chelatedmin.com/index-3.html

[3] *www.nhs.uk/Livewell/workplacehealth/Pages/energyslumps.aspx*

[4] *https://www.ncbi.nlm.nih.gov/pubmed/8184963*

[5] *http://news.bbc.co.uk/1/hi/health/4616603.stm*

[6] *https://www.ncbi.nlm.nih.gov/pubmed/26043918*

[7] *www.medicinenet.com/small_intestinal_bacterial_overgrowth/ article.htm*

[8] *https://www.theibsnetwork.org/diet/fodmaps/*

[9] *Foodpsychology.cornell.edu/research/biasing-health-halos*

[10] *Thinkmoney.co.uk/news-advice/are-you-wasting-money-on-an-unused-gym-membership*

[11] *https://www.statista.com/statistics/241683/nikes-sales-worldwide-since-2004/*

[12] *www.worldometers.info/weight-loss*

[13] *http://sportsmedicine.about.com/cs/injuries/a/doms.htm*

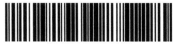

Printed in Great Britain
by Amazon